The Language of the Soul in Narrative Therapy

The Language of the Soul in Narrative Therapy uniquely bridges the gap between narrative therapy and spirituality to describe how the theory and practice of narrative therapy may be expanded and enriched by incorporating the language of the soul.

Divided into three parts, the book begins by contextualizing the approach of narrative therapy and spirituality. Chapters then debate the complexity of the 'soul' as a term drawing on the work of Christian mystics and philosophers, such as Teresa of Avila, Edith Stein, Merleau-Ponty, and Bakhtin, to show how their theoretical ideas can be incorporated in counseling practice and spiritual direction. The book concludes by discussing how the language of the soul can be integrated and applied in postmodern practice.

With case examples from faith belief systems, such as Christianity, Buddhism, Paganism, Wicca, and Yazidism, throughout, this book is essential reading for therapists, clinical social workers, and counselors in practice and graduate training, as well as spiritual directors and pastoral counselors interested in the ideas and practices of narrative therapy.

Laura Béres, MSW, MA, PhD, is an academic and clinical social worker, writing in the areas of narrative therapy, spirituality, and critical reflection on practice.

With contributions from:
David Crawley, MSc, MTh, PGDipCouns, PhD, is a practical theologian and spiritual direction educator. His current writing focuses on narrative approaches to spiritual care.

The Language of the Soul in Narrative Therapy

Spirituality in Clinical Theory and Practice

Laura Béres
with contributions from David Crawley

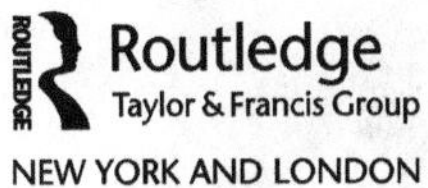

NEW YORK AND LONDON

Cover image: © Getty Images

First published 2023
by Routledge
605 Third Avenue, New York, NY 10158

and by Routledge
4 Park Square, Milton Park, Abingdon, Oxon, OX14 4RN

Routledge is an imprint of the Taylor & Francis Group, an informa business

Library of Congress Cataloguing-in-Publication Data
Names: Béres, Laura, author.
Title: The language of the soul in narrative therapy : spirituality in clinical theory and practice / Laura Béres; with contributions from David Crawley.
Description: New York, NY : Routledge, 2022. | Includes bibliographical references and index.
Identifiers: LCCN 2021062877 (print) | LCCN 2021062878 (ebook) | ISBN 9780367678081 (hardback) | ISBN 9780367684228 (paperback) | ISBN 9781003137450 (ebook)
Subjects: LCSH: Narrative therapy. | Spirituality. | Psychotherapy.
Classification: LCC RC489.S74 B47 2022 (print) | LCC RC489.S74 (ebook) | DDC 616.89/165--dc23/eng/20220125
LC record available at https://lccn.loc.gov/2021062877
LC ebook record available at https://lccn.loc.gov/2021062878

ISBN: 978-0-367-67808-1 (hbk)
ISBN: 978-0-367-68422-8 (pbk)
ISBN: 978-1-003-13745-0 (ebk)

DOI: 10.4324/9781003137450

Typeset in Bembo
by MPS Limited, Dehradun

Contents

Acknowledgments

Laura Béres

I want to begin by acknowledging the influence on my thinking of Louise Nelstrop, Barnabas Palfrey, and Peter Tyler, whom I met through Sarum College in Salisbury, England. I am particularly grateful to Peter Tyler for his support as I completed a thesis under his guidance. I have referenced Louise's and Peter's work many times in this book and am indebted to their rigorous academic study in the area of spirituality and mysticism.

I am grateful to my colleagues at King's University College at Western University in London, Canada, and their encouragement of my highly interdisciplinary areas of interest.

I want to also acknowledge how much I learn every time I am in a therapeutic conversation with someone and wish to thank everyone who has shared their journey with me in this context. I have changed names and identifying details as I have described my therapeutic work in this book, but I believe their souls still shine through and enrich this work.

I am thankful that David Crawley was willing to contribute a chapter to this book and engage in a concluding dialogue in the final chapter, enriching this book all the more.

Finally, I am grateful to my husband, David, and son, Liam, for all their support and unwavering belief in my ability to pursue my interests and complete this book.

Introduction

Laura Béres and David Crawley

Laura's Introduction of Herself and the Story of This Book

Iexperienced an evocative nighttime dream early on in the process of writing this book. In the dream, I was attending an academic conference with some of my most highly respected colleagues and friends. I was anxiously attempting to make sure that I would be able to create the opportunity to have a meal and a chat with each of them over the course of the conference. At one point in the dream, having managed to coordinate a convenient time, I was meeting with a colleague who was giving me a foot massage. (I would like to point out this has never happened in any actual conference I have attended!) I looked down in my dream and was horrified to realize how dirty my feet were after a day of walking about in sandals, and so I suggested I go wash my feet before continuing. Then, as happens in dreams, I found myself in a different setting – in a huge artist's loft-style apartment where a cat had caught and killed several pregnant mice, leaving a sad and unpleasant mess for me to clean up. I went to ask my partner for help, but he was busy wrapping his head in strips of linen to make a mask, and he asked why I was not singing from the script I was holding. I said I would read any parts from the script to assist him in preparing for his performance, but I was not going to sing. Finally, back at the conference, I reassured another worried conference attendee that she did not need to be embarrassed about having missed an unexpected rehearsal since the actress from *Titanic* (Kate Winslet, but I could not remember her name in my dream) had stepped in and filled the necessary role. Nonetheless, I pored over the details of the rest of the conference to ensure we would not miss any other important meetings.

One of my colleagues, in my waking life, recently mentioned Thomas Moore's *Care of the Soul* (2016) and given my interest in the language of the soul, I quickly bought it and read it with much relish. In it, Moore suggests that we should not attempt to intellectually interpret our dreams but rather consider what the more soulful and artistic aspects of ourselves might be attempting to communicate. When I considered this dream I have

DOI: 10.4324/9781003137450-1

described, it initially seemed rich with worry and advice as I began the process of writing this book. I could make a rational connection between the colleagues in the dream and realizing how many of my respected colleagues and friends have had a great impact on my thinking regarding narrative therapy, spirituality, and the language of the soul and how I hoped to spend the appropriate time and space to properly honor each of their contributions in this book. At the same time, I wondered if my dream was showing me that I was worrying about not being quite ready for the task involved in writing this book. My feet were, and still are, metaphorically grubby. Having considered this further I have come to think this does not need to be a bad thing. Perhaps my dirty feet show that I am firmly planted on the ground, doing the work of offering counseling to people and listening to their stories, as well as intrigued by the writing of philosophers and mystics. My first reaction to the dream was that I needed to clean everything – my feet and the mess left in the loft-style apartment – before being ready to even begin this book, let alone finish it. Yet, being open to other ways of considering the dream, I wondered if it might also contain a warning not to kill creativity and artistic expression through worries about everything needing to be just so. I hope readers will be willing to engage with the ideas and reflections in this book with an openness to the possibilities about the language of the soul, which will be influenced by philosophers and mystics who might seem quite ethereal at times, but which I have attempted to keep grounded in practice experience. This project of writing about the language of the soul has come about over many years, having been influenced by many strands of varying types of inquiry and reflective practice, and as a postmodern narrative therapist I do not consider the ideas I will share in this book as a whole and single or static 'Truth'. Hence, these ideas might seem messy. I hope readers will also be willing to engage in this complexity. Nonetheless, in order to be transparent about the position from which I am writing, I will start here by describing my background and how I have come to be writing this book now.

I grew up in England, moving to Canada as a teen and so completing the last year of high school in what felt like a very new context, prior to beginning my undergraduate university degree in Psychology. I mention that I grew up in England, because I still feel very much influenced by those early years in English culture. After completing my BA, I worked in group homes for a few years and volunteered in various settings prior to completing my master's degree in Social Work. I was then able to begin employment in a Catholic family counseling agency where I worked for the next 15 years. I had not been raised within the Roman Catholic tradition and worked with very few service users who identified as Roman Catholic, but the faith-based traditions of the agency seeped into a good portion of the clinical supervision I received in a very reflective rather than impositional manner. I loved working with all the various people I met in counseling sessions there, and I was particularly inspired by the women,

men, and children who were responding to the effects of trauma in their lives and moving toward their preferred ways of living. During this time, a woman who was living with a man who had used abusive behaviors toward her many times mentioned to me that she was reading romance novels to attempt to learn how to behave like the heroines in the novels in the hopes that this would protect her from further beatings. I worked with her, deconstructing and reflecting upon these ideas, but this also led to my interest in pursuing my PhD in Education, within a focus on Critical Pedagogy and Cultural Studies. I was curious about how people were negotiating and learning from the messages presented in popular cultural discourses, which was an area of study that had not been incorporated into my previous social work education. I continued to work part-time in the same counseling agency while I completed my course work and research. It was during this time that I first attended a weeklong workshop presented by Michael White and was introduced to narrative therapy practices and ideas. The whole approach of providing scaffolding (inspired by the work of educational psychologist Lev Vygotsky) for externalizing conversations was particularly helpful as I contemplated the manner in which some people might also be using popular cultural texts as a framework, or scaffold, to attempt to make sense of their situations. I was also interested in how it might be possible to assist people in externalizing internalized discourses, like those which romanticize abuse within many popular cultural texts. It was a wonderful time, learning about Foucault, Gramsci, Freire, to name a few, in my doctoral studies, while continuing to work in direct practice, and at the same time being excited by the possibilities of how Michael White was bringing a range of philosophical, cognitive psychological, and cultural anthropological ideas into the ongoing development of narrative therapy practices.

Having completed my PhD, I was torn between remaining in direct practice full-time or pursuing an academic position. I decided that since I so enjoyed and valued counseling within the profession of Social Work that I would like to be involved in contributing to the field of Social Work by teaching future social workers, and so moved into a university position. I have now been teaching Social Work direct practice courses, including a narrative therapy course, for 18 years in a publicly funded Roman Catholic liberal arts university. I did not search out a Catholic university as a place to teach. I was drawn to this university due to the excellent reputation of their School of Social Work, but I have appreciated the smaller size and nature of a liberal arts university, the respect for spirituality and all faith traditions, and the encouragement of the teacher-scholar model within this context. However, that is certainly not the end of the story. It was only after I took up this academic position that I was able to pursue training at the Dulwich Centre, and so enrolled in one of the seven-month training courses offered there at the time. The course was made up of two block periods of study in Adelaide with Michael White and his colleagues, David Denborough,

Shona Russel, Maggie Carey, and Caroline Mackey. Between each block of study in Adelaide, I was engaged in reflective practice, recording counseling sessions and sending reflections to the Dulwich Centre instructors for feedback. During this time, I also worked alongside Michael and some of my Canadian narrative therapy colleagues, including Jim Duvall and Scot Copper, in a narrative outsider witness community practice context. In this context, we worked alongside Indigenous and non-Indigenous people in Southwestern Ontario in response to community conflict regarding land rights. Shortly after that, I then had the opportunity to attend a follow-up intensive training session with Michael in Adelaide a few short months before his untimely death early in 2008.

It is difficult at times to recall the exact timing and sequence of the various events that have occurred but alongside the development of my narrative practices I was also becoming increasingly interested in spirituality, mindfulness, and critical reflection on practice. I began expanding the traditional bio-psycho-social assessment model to also include 'spiritual' in my own writing and also in class with Social Work students. I had first been introduced to critical reflection, and critical social theory through my doctoral work, mindfulness was becoming more and more of interest to practitioners everywhere, and I became curious about the similarities between mindfulness, with its Buddhist underpinnings, other contemplative practices in Christian and Hindu traditions, and critical reflection.

Another strand of my story, which has had an ongoing impact, started during my first year-long sabbatical when I traveled to Iona, in the Scottish Hebrides, and began learning about Celtic spirituality and Celtic Christianity. Iona has been described as a 'thin place', which is a term used within the literature regarding Celtic spirituality, to refer to a place where the boundary between this and the other world is thin and so can be experienced as more spiritual. I decided to audit an academic course about Celtic spirituality which was offered as part of an MA in Christian Spirituality in England. What I particularly appreciate about Celtic spirituality is its close relation to Indigenous spiritualities, with a consideration of the spark of the Divine in all living beings, a love and respect of nature and creativity, and the link to monastic contemplative traditions. That is a rather sweeping overgeneralization, perhaps, but certainly my earliest writing about Celtic spirituality stressed the spiritual connection between people and physical places (Béres, 2012; 2013; 2017). Later, I also wrote about my pilgrimage along St. Cuthbert's Way in Scotland and Northern England, and the link between walking in nature, mindful or contemplative practices, and my ongoing attempt to integrate ideas of simplicity and pilgrimage into everyday travel (Béres, 2018). These ideas regarding the need for simplicity had actually started earlier on social justice educational trips I was involved in with students. For several years in a row, I traveled with students from Canada to the Cuernavaca Centre for Intercultural Dialogue and Development in Mexico, where we all learned about the impact of the northern hemisphere's lifestyle on the made-poor of Mexico. I have traveled with students to remote fly-in Indigenous communities in Canada, and also to India and China where the focus of these experiential learning courses was the recognition of the range of various cultures and various ways of considering the role of Social Work across cultures. Students would return from these trips never again being able to think theirs was the only way of doing things, learning from other cultures rather than imposing their Canadian Social Work lens on to another. Each of these trips involved an element of pilgrimage as I also learned about other cultures, became more aware of some of the taken-for-granted assumptions within my own cultural context, and, perhaps oddly, recommitted each time to a greater wish for simplicity.

It was helpful, as my interest in yet a fourth academic discipline was continuing to percolate, to learn from the experts in this fields of Celtic and Christian spirituality. I was hooked after auditing the first course and went on to enroll and complete the MA in Christian Spirituality Much like the training at the Dulwich Centre, this course of study required my attendance at week-long blocks of classes as well as involvement in remote feedback. My final thesis which I completed in fulfillment of the degree requirements was regarding the contributions of Teresa of Avila and Edith Stein in considering conceptions of the soul for narrative therapy. I continue to consider myself a narrative therapist and find my philosophical and political values closely align with narrative practices. Yet, as my interest in spirituality, and my own contemplative practices, continued to develop, I began to realize that the underlying theories of narrative therapy did not provide any method for conceptualizing the soul, which is important for many service users and providers. I had always defined spirituality in very broad terms which included the idea of it providing people with a sense of meaning and purpose. I could integrate conversations about spirituality in therapeutic conversations as people spoke of their values, hopes, and dreams, but I wanted to think through how to engage with ideas of the soul without a full-blown sense of dissonance – or to use a less medical-model word: discombobulation! This book, therefore, has come about in response to my wish to explore what has felt like a little bit of a 'gap' in the theory of narrative therapy, building upon the foundational work I completed in my most recent MA thesis. Yet, I have also expanded the focus on Teresa of Avila and Edith Stein to include contributions from Merleau-Ponty, and a description of how critical reflection and contemplative practices have been integrated into my approach to studying these philosophers and my own therapeutic and spiritual practices. Finally, I have invited David Crawley to write a chapter regarding the contributions of Bakhtin as they relate to narrative and spiritual practices. Before David introduces himself, I will first clarify how my interest in spiritual direction came about and how I distinguish between counseling, or therapy, which discusses spirituality, spiritual direction, and pastoral counseling.

As someone who describes herself as an introvert, I am a person who appreciates being able to attend silent retreats. My first experience was with a weekend silent Buddhist retreat. It was in a beautiful rural setting, with wonderful vegetarian meals provided, and facilitated sitting, lying, standing, and walking meditations. One problem for me was that I was assigned to a shared bedroom with someone who snored very loudly all night, and I had not brought earplugs with me, so it was not quite as silent as I would have liked. I continued to crave the experience of a silent retreat and while immersed in the final writing stages of my PhD dissertation, a family friend and Anglican priest suggested I might appreciate staying in the guesthouse at the convent of the Sisters of St. John the Divine. I had never even visited a convent before, and found the silence exceptionally refreshing. It helped that all guests are provided with a single private bedroom. The convent is founded within a Benedictine monastic tradition, with the sisters living in silence for the majority of the time. However, once each week they have a 'talking dinner' where there is a lot of chatter, and they speak and sing in their worship services, as well as in the workshops and spiritual direction they offer. I found my time at the convent so refreshing that I have returned many times but have only ever managed to stay for weekend retreats. However, three years ago, having been introduced to the ideas of Ignatian spiritual direction during my MA in Christian Spirituality, I attended my first eight-day silent retreat at a local Ignatian Centre. Although the whole eight days was primarily in silence, I met with a spiritual director for one hour of discussion each day, and it was also possible to attend worship services in which there was speaking and singing. The Ignatian Centre is set within hundreds of acres of land, with forest, and gardens, and labyrinths, allowing for a great deal of the silent time being able to be enjoyed outside. I found this such a lovely rejuvenating time and the process of spiritual direction so useful that I decided I wanted to pursue the Ignatian Spiritual Exercises. These were originally designed to be completed during a 30-day silent retreat, but it is possible to pursue them in what is termed the 19th annotation. This refers to the 19th 'note' within the original exercises which suggests that those people who cannot remove themselves from their ordinary day to day commitments to conduct a 30-day retreat may pursue the exercises by engaging in one hour of silent prayer/meditation each day and by meeting with an appropriately trained spiritual director once each week; This is what I did, completing the exercises over approximately nine months. My hope, in the future, is to attend the Ignatian Centre for further training in spiritual direction so that I may offer spiritual direction as well as counseling services. This interest involved needing to sort out my own thoughts about what the differences are between spiritual direction, counseling, which might include the area of spirituality, and a third professional discipline: pastoral counseling. These three different disciplinary professional practices could probably be represented in a Venn diagram, with each represented as a circle which overlaps with another and them all overlapping in the center. Nonetheless, I will attempt to describe some of the main general differences between these practices.

I have come to consider spirituality as an area to be inquired into as one element of a person's life in a counseling or Social Work assessment. Spirituality can be a resource and bolster resilience, but spirituality and religion may also have caused pain in a person's life and so the person may be wishing to heal from some pain and trauma related to this. So, in counseling, spirituality is not the main focus of work or conversation but is part of it as appropriate to the person requesting services. However, many counselors do not feel adequately prepared to engage in useful conversations about a person's faith or spirituality and so would be inclined to refer someone to their religious faith community leader to discuss such topics should they arise. On the other hand, spiritual direction is focused primarily on the person's spirituality, and their relationship to the Divine, or God. A person may seek spiritual direction in order to deepen their ongoing spiritual practices, or because they wish toaccess support as they are discerning the next steps in their lives. Spiritual directors may not be qualified as therapists and, if not, would refer those seeking direction to counselors if mental health issues surface within their spiritual direction conversations. Finally, although a further over-simplification, pastoral counseling combines theology and traditional counseling approaches and so could be considered as drawing upon both counseling and pastoral care practices. Pastoral counseling in its earliest forms would have been provided by pastors, or people with religious qualifications and ministries, working out of church communities, but linked to hospitals and other mental and physical health settings. In the early days of this profession, pastors would have had very few courses in counseling theories or practices and most of their interactions with people would have been based upon their theological understandings. The discipline has grown and developed and there are specific training programs now for people wishing to become pastoral counselors. Nonetheless, it is useful to highlight that pastoral counselors continue to be influenced by theology as well as Psychology, or counseling practices.

Traditionally, narrative therapy has not articulated the role of spirituality and the language of the soul in its theory and practice, and I believe it can benefit from considering these aspects. There are some narrative therapists already incorporating spirituality and faith, but there has been no theorizing of the language of the soul. Also traditionally, spiritual direction and pastoral counseling would have been influenced most by Freudian or Jungian psychological theories. It is refreshing to see that there are some more recent exceptions to this, and a handful of academics and practitioners are finding that narrative therapy practices offer much, particularly if they are committed to liberation and feminist theologies. I am hoping within this book that I will offer ideas that will further bridge and encourage discussion across these areas of narrative therapy, spiritual direction, and pastoral counseling.

At long last, I invite David Crawley to introduce himself.

David's Introduction of Himself

I am thrilled to have the opportunity to make a modest contribution to this book. Studying narrative therapy in the early 2000s ignited a desire for narrative therapy and spirituality to get to know one another better. When I asked Google who might share this hope, just one name emerged: Laura Béres. Her books on narrative practice and spirituality were yet to be written, but I found articles which reflected a heart on a spiritual quest and a mind keen to integrate this with postmodern practice (Béres, 2004; 2012). It was some years before I met Laura in person. New Zealand is a long way from Canada, and I was preoccupied with completing my doctoral studies, which had me immersed in Foucault and discourse analysis. But let me go back a few steps.

I am a fourth-generation New Zealander, descended from English and Scottish immigrants. My interest in spirituality began before I can remember, as our family faithfully attended the Presbyterian church in each small town in which we lived. Cutting a long story (including a career as a mathematics teacher) short, this led eventually to theological study and a teaching position in an ecumenical theological college, where I still teach on a part-time basis. Critical to this part of my story is a period in which I found myself in a spiritual wilderness. After completing my studies, I theoretically knew more than ever about God, but experientially I felt dry and adrift. A colleague who was beginning to explore contemplative spirituality suggested that spiritual direction or a silent retreat might be helpful. I decided to try both. I booked a weekend in a Catholic retreat center, run by the Sisters of Mercy, where my retreat was guided by one of the sisters. There was no dramatic epiphany, but this experience marked a gentle beginning to a journey out of the wilderness and into a more contemplative form of spirituality. Not many years later, I completed training as a spiritual director in the Christian tradition, and my theological teaching focused increasingly on spirituality and pastoral care.

For Laura, narrative ideas and practice preceded the exploration of spirituality. My experience was the reverse. As Laura has indicated, there are times when a person seeking spiritual guidance may also need the help of a professional counselor or psychologist. But there are also occasions, found in the overlap between spiritual direction and counseling, when a spiritual director with sufficient training and competence can journey safely with a person in distress. My need to grow in both confidence and competence in that zone prompted me to pursue counseling training. Initially this involved exposure to person-centered therapy and transactional analysis. I found the grounding in person-centered attitudes and skills helpful.

From theological and spiritual perspectives, however, some of the ideas underpinning these approaches felt thin. Little or no attention was given at that time to notions such as relationality, justice, and ethical purpose, which, in my own tradition, call people beyond mere self-realization.

Without quite knowing what I was getting into, I then began post-graduate study in narrative therapy, at the University of Waikato, in New Zealand. My tutors were intrigued that a person of faith was choosing to immerse himself in the most postmodern of therapeutic programs! Yet it was in this context that I found what had earlier been missing – an approach to therapy which wanted to think about power, truth claims, social justice, relationality, and hope. People connected with the university had produced a book called *Narrative Therapy in Practice: An Archaeology of Hope* (Monk, Winslade, Crocket, & Epston, 1997). The metaphor works as well for spiritual direction as it does for counseling. Not only were there resonances here with my own spirituality, but I found the teaching of this 'secular' program respectful toward, and inclusive of, Indigenous (Māori) spirituality. I recall a visiting professor from the United Kingdom remarking on how often spirituality was mentioned in our class discussions, given the postmodern basis of the program. There was even a blessing spoken before food was shared. For those familiar with the Indigenous culture of this land, this was not an oddity. The visitor's point was that spirituality, like any discourse, must be open to critical reflection, and this was a given. In fact, it was discovering the work of Foucault, via Michael White and our own teachers, which led to my doctoral research, in which I applied Foucauldian discourse analysis to narratives of resistance to religious authority.

Alongside these positive experiences, I was also aware of the tensions which exist between ideas which circulated in my spiritual direction context, such as the notion of the 'true self', and the social constructionist framework of narrative therapy. I continued to wrestle with these questions over the years and later developed some of the ideas which are included in my chapter in this book. In 2016, I attended my first conference of the (then) British Association for the Study of Spirituality, in Manchester, England, and was delighted to see Laura's name on the list of delegates and presenters. I was even more pleased when I was able to chat briefly with her about her work and some of the issues that were exercising my thinking. Since then, through emails and personal conversation at a subsequent conference, I learned something of her own ongoing journey of integration, which she has described above.

It is exciting to see this integrative process coming to another stage of fruition in the work of this book, which I view as a work of hospitality. In it, Laura has furnished a broad table at which interesting guests may be met and a diversity of voices heard. Here, practitioners of all kinds for whom the soul matters are bound to find both personal and professional nourishment. Thank you, Laura, for your generous hospitality, and for the privilege of helping in a small way to set the table.

References

Béres, L. (2004). A reflective journey: Spirituality and postmodern practice. *Currents: New Scholarship in the Human Services*, *3*(1).

Béres, L. (2012). A thin place: Narratives of space and place, Celtic spirituality and meaning. *Journal of Religion and Spirituality in Social Work: Social Thought*, *31*(4), 394–413.

Béres, L. (2013). Celtic spirituality and postmodern geography: Narratives of engagement with place. *Journal for the Study of Spirituality*, *2*(2), 170–185.

Béres, L. (2017). Celtic spirituality: Exploring the fascination across time and place. In B. Crisp (Ed.). *The Routledge Handbook of Religion, Spirituality, and Social Work* (pp. 100–107). Routledge.

Béres, L. (2018). How travel might become more like pilgrimage: An auto-ethnographic study. *Journal for the Study of Spirituality*, *8*(2), 160–172.

Monk, G., Winslade, J., Crocket, K., & Epston, D. (Eds). (1997). *Narrative therapy in practice: The archaeology of hope*. Jossey-Bass.

Moore, T. (2016). *Care of the soul: A guide for cultivating depth and sacredness in everyday life, twenty-fifth anniversary edition*. Harper Perennial.

Part I

The Context and Approach: Narrative Therapy and Spirituality

1 The Self/Identity in Narrative Therapy

Laura Béres

Lydia[1] telephoned the counseling agency in which I work part time and specifically asked in her initial request for services that she be able to meet with me for individual counseling. Once I was able to offer an appointment, Lydia's intake information was forwarded to me and I read that she described herself as 'experiencing anxiety and wanting to deal with some past issues'. There was no indication as to why she had asked to meet with me in particular, although I assumed it was because she knew I identified as a narrative therapist or due to my interest in, and respect for, others' spirituality. I started my first meeting with Lydia as I do most first appointments, asking her to tell me a little bit about what was going well in her life and what the supports and resources were in her life that had been helping her cope with the problem she wanted to discuss while she had been waiting for us to be able to meet. I explained that I preferred to start like this, if she did not mind, because then when she did talk about the problem(s) she was wanting to discuss we would be better able to consider them within her broader context. She agreed to this approach and described her happy home situation with her husband, her 9-year-old son, and her 12-year old daughter. She described a good network of friends and a happy upbringing with loving parents. She said her mother had often been rather anxious and the sort of parent who would tell her not to swim too far out in the lake or climb too high since she might not make it back to shore or she might fall and hurt herself. She commented that this could have been the start of her own anxiety. She also indicated that her parents were churchgoers and expected her to also attend regularly with them. She described herself as always having been a good rule-follower and having continued to regularly attend church until very recently. However, she said she was now fed up with listening to 'white middle-aged men preaching at her', and found herself anxious while in church, but also anxious about not wanting to go to church anymore. As we discussed her situation further, Lydia went on to describe her spiritual life as being extremely important to her despite her frustration with the church she continued to attend from time to time. She spoke of her belief in a transcendent or divine being, her comfort with mystery, and her need to feed her soul somehow – she said walking in

DOI: 10.4324/9781003137450-3

nature often helped with this need. Through this discussion, she also mentioned I had been recommended as a counselor for her due to my interest in spirituality. As we brought our first meeting to a close, I checked with her as to whether she felt the focus of our discussion had been okay with her, or whether she felt any frustration in not having talked more about the anxiety yet. She said this had been a useful conversation, and I added that, to use a phrase I had heard Michael White use many times, 'problems dissolve' often when we focus on articulating those areas in a person's life which are rich with meaning-making and personal values.

As a narrative therapist, I could have approached Lydia's story and her 'presenting problem' of anxiety in a number of different ways. I could have been curious about her story of herself and her relationship with anxiety over the years, in order to assist her in moving from a problem saturated story to a preferred story, or I could have assisted her in externalizing anxiety, characterizing it richly, and examining its effects in her life for her then to evaluate and consider. We could have examined the power and impact of religious discourses that were now frustrating her, externalizing those messages that had been internalized, or even engaging in an "absent but implicit" (White, 2007a) conversation where her complaints about the 'middle-aged men preaching at her' could be considered in terms of what she was now standing up against and what that implied she holds dear. What caught my attention the most was her wish to feed her soul.

As I described in the Introduction, I have considered myself a narrative therapist for many years and have been committed to writing about and teaching narrative therapy for almost as long (Béres, 2010; 2014; 2017a; Béres & Page Nichols, 2010; Duvall & Béres, 2007; 2011). Indeed, narrative therapy continues to be my preferred way of interacting with others in counseling and community practice settings, but as my personal and research interests have expanded to include a fascination with spirituality (Béres, 2012; 2013; 2016; 2017b; Rogers & Béres, 2017), and particularly with the mystics' writing about spirituality, I have begun to experience what is best described as a 'gap' within narrative therapy's theory and practice. Rather than continuing to explore these two areas, narrative therapy and spirituality, as two separate and distinct interests, or to merely attempt to fit conversations about spirituality into narrative therapy practices (see chapter 7 in Béres, 2014 or Rogers & Béres, 2017), my aim for this book is to broaden the theoretical base of narrative therapy to include discussions of the complex ways in which the soul can be understood. Some narrative therapists may conflate the soul with notions regarding a 'core self' and thereby refute the language of the soul as being too structured, on the one hand, or too religious, on the other, but the literature regarding the soul suggests a complexity and fluidity that may fit comfortably within postmodern therapies.

Narrative therapy, as a postmodern and social constructionist approach, has purposefully moved away from the images of 'depth' and 'core' in regard to people, and rather has focused on the image of 'text' and the effects on people's lives of how they construct their identities through the stories they tell about themselves to themselves and to others. This includes an awareness of the power of discourses to which they have access, and which will often influence the storying of their identities (Béres, 1999; 2002; White, 1995). This approach focuses, therefore, on the fluidity of identity and possibility for change and learning, rather than on structures of the self or expectations for normative behaviors.

Narrative therapists engage with people from a stance of curiosity, asking people how they make meaning of events, what their preferences for themselves would be, what their hopes and dreams are, and what would provide a sense of meaning and purpose. Since spirituality within therapeutic practice literature is often described as that which gives meaning and purpose to someone's life (Canda, 1988; Cook, Powell & Sims, 2009; Crisp, 2010), I believe narrative practices can easily open up space for people to have conversations about spirituality.

From as early as Plato (428–347 BCE) philosophers have considered the soul and pondered the relationship between the soul and the Divine (Tyler, 2016). Although Western postmodern therapists might argue that ideas about the soul have been structured by organized religion, and Christianity in particular, these were areas of curiosity well before the Christian Era. In fact, some of these discourses will be described and traced over time in chapter three. As present-day academic disciplines such as psychology, psychotherapy, and social work, and the associated professional practices, have attempted to present themselves as 'rigorous and scientific' they have also attempted to distance themselves from religion. This has had the unfortunate consequence of also distancing themselves from spirituality and any consideration of the soul, although there have been a few notable exceptions (Hillman, 2007; Moore, 2016; Peck, 2003; Tyler, 2016). I would like to reintroduce these topics into the literature regarding narrative therapy in order to broaden the conversations possible within narrative practices. I believe this will not only facilitate a richer range of conversations about religious faith and spirituality, which are important for true cultural humility in our practices, but will also underscore the usefulness and appropriateness of narrative practices for spiritual directors and pastoral counselors. There are a handful of spiritual directors and pastoral counselors already using narrative practices and I will discuss their contributions later in this chapter.

To begin, I will describe the development of narrative therapy and its theoretical underpinnings. I will then describe what I mean by a 'gap' in narrative therapy's theory, drawing upon work by Guilfoyle (2014) and Schwartz (1999) who have also indicated they have experienced something as missing in narrative therapy's practice and theory. Schwartz particularly suggests that concepts such as spirituality and the soul are absent from narrative therapy's understanding, while Guilfoyle points to inconsistencies but ultimately continues to rely on post-structuralists' theories to address these concerns. Although post-structuralists might argue the language of the soul is merely another social discourse needing to be deconstructed, I agree with Schwartz that practice experience suggests that there is more to people than only socially constructed identities. I also suggest that many of the people who consult with us will use the language of the soul, just as Lydia did, and so it is sensible to think through the possibilities of this language.

The Beginnings of Narrative Therapy Theory and Practice

Narrative therapy, or 'narrative practice' as it is often referred to since it can be used in both psychotherapy and community practice contexts, is commonly described as being a relatively new and postmodern approach to practice. Yet it is also more recently being described as one of the most popular and mainstream approaches to counseling and social work. Blanton (2005) has gone so far as to say it "has quickly become the leading approach to family therapy" (p. 69).

Although there are many narrative practice training centers around the world, the Dulwich Centre in Australia, which Michael and Cheryl White opened in 1983, is probably most often thought of as the primary center for teaching narrative therapy and community work skills, and this is where I received the majority of my training in narrative therapy. Cheryl White and David Denborough have also been instrumental in the development of the first MA program in Narrative Therapy and Community Practice which the Dulwich Centre offers in conjunction with the University of Melbourne. David Epston, as the co-originator of narrative therapy with Michael White, was also the co-founder, with Johnella Bird, of The Family Therapy Centre which opened in New Zealand in 1988, and he has worked closely with the Dulwich Centre since Michael White's death in 2008.

White and Epston's first book regarding narrative ways of working was initially published by Dulwich Centre publications in 1989 entitled *Literary Means to Therapeutic Ends* and then re-published as *Narrative Means to Therapeutic Ends* by W. W. Norton in 1990. Although White had begun influencing social work and family therapy practice in Australia earlier in academic journal format (White, 1984), this publication could be considered the first narrative therapy book to reach beyond Australia and New Zealand and begin to influence family therapy, counseling, and social work practices in the rest of the world.

In "Story, Knowledge and Power", the introductory chapter of the seminal work *Narrative Means to Therapeutic Ends* (1990), White begins by describing the influences on himself and Epston as they were developing their approach to practice. As he also points out in a later interview (White, 1995), he and Epston were both avid readers outside of their discipline of social work, being very much influenced by anthropology, philosophy, and educational and cognitive psychology. White points out that it was Gregory Bateson's work that introduced him to social scientists' fascination with how people interpret and make meaning of their worlds. Bateson challenged the usefulness of linear causality and proposed that people make meaning of events based on the context in which they receive those events, "that is, by the network of premises and presuppositions that constitute our maps of the world" (White & Epston, 1990, p. 2). Developing their theories while immersed in the world of family therapy in the 1970s, much of White and Epston's theorizing was in reaction to what they saw not working in therapy and wanting to intervene differently. White explains, for example, that Bateson's interpretive method,

> rather than proposing that some underlying structure or dysfunction in the family determines the behavior and interactions of family members, would propose that it is the meaning that members attribute to events that determines their behavior. Thus, for some considerable time I have been interested in how persons organize their lives around specific meanings and how, in so doing, they inadvertently contribute to the 'survival' of, as well as the 'career' of, the problem.
>
> (White & Epston, 1990, p. 3)

This gives an example of what continues to be of most importance to narrative therapists: a movement away from considering underlying structures or internal dysfunctions and toward a privileging of people's meaning-making behaviors. Drawing upon Victor Turner and Edward Bruner's work, as well as Erving Goffman's and Clifford Geertz', White and Epston describe how the 'positivist physical sciences', 'biological sciences', and various approaches within 'social sciences' use varying analogies or metaphors which then have an impact on how problems and solutions are constructed. Wishing to move away from metaphors of machines or organisms, which would then focus on attempting to find the cause of a problem and then have an 'expert' attempt to correct it, they were more interested in the analogy of text. Using an analogy of life as a text, problems could be considered a performance of a dominant or problem storyline and the way forward out of that problem storyline would involve assisting people in re-authoring life events and stepping into preferred storylines (White & Epston, 1990).

White (2005) has also remarked that he believed psychotherapy had begun to overly privilege emotions in therapeutic conversations, whereas he and Epston were much more interested in privileging how people made meaning of events. This can lead to an accusation that narrative therapy ignores feelings, but it rather assists people in discussing feelings in a different way. White has suggested, for example, that it can be more therapeutically beneficial when someone is crying to ask, 'If you could take one of those tears and open it up, what might be inside it?' rather than, 'Tell me how you are feeling'. The former question does not ignore the emotion, but rather invites the person to be curious about it. The latter statement of direction is more apt to result in frustration since it is obvious what is being felt, or may result in a reinforcement of the emotion. White and Epston did not focus on emotions in their narrative practices but this does not mean they did not believe emotions existed. Perhaps the same could be said for the soul.

Moving on to explore the effects of Michel Foucault's thought on knowledge and power, which continues to be considered a fundamental aspect of narrative practice, White describes Foucault as suggesting "we are subject to power through normalizing 'truths' that shape our lives and relationships" (White & Epston, 1990, p. 19) and that,

> when discussing 'truths', Foucault is subscribing not to the belief that there exist objective or intrinsic facts about the nature of persons but instead to constructed ideas that are accorded a truth status. These 'truths' are 'normalizing' in the sense they construct norms around which persons are incited to shape or constitute their lives.
>
> (White & Epston, 1990, pp. 19–20)

This, I believe, is often misinterpreted in therapy circles as suggesting that as postmodern therapists we are encouraged to believe in multiple truths as if they each contained equal worth, which can lead to an accusation of relativism within narrative therapy. However, whenever I heard White respond to such an accusation in a training context (2006) he would clarify that he was suggesting not that everything should go without question but, rather, that nothing should go without question, arguing that ideas are accorded labels of truth due to certain discourses that support that status. For instance, many of Freud's concepts have taken on the status of 'truths' rather than being considered ideas influenced by one possible theoretical view. In a postmodern practice setting, this results in examining with people the influence of discourses and the elements of those discourses which support a certain idea as being true (e.g., discourses of masculinity which suggest 'boys will be boys').

Seemingly anticipating future questions raised by Guilfoyle (2014), White says,

> [I]n making the point that our lives are embraced by the private but constructed stories that we have about life, I've perhaps been a little too emphatic. If the idea that stories "live us" or "embrace our lives" leads to the notion that persons go about life rather mindlessly re-enacting or reproducing these stories, then I think that is a problematic idea. Stories provide the frames that make it possible for us to interpret our experience, and these acts of interpretation are achievements that we take an active part in.
>
> (White, 1995, p. 15)

In this way, White raises something which Guilfoyle (2014) later suggests is an inconsistency within narrative therapy's theoretical base: if a sense of self/identity is socially constructed, how can there also be an element of a person able to be active in resisting those discourses and dominant storylines? However, White was, at the same time as he was discussing the power of discourses, also saying that text is just one analogy and that although stories are powerfully constitutive, people are also active agents in their lives rather than merely docile and duped by discourse. He says that no single possible story can be free of contradictions and ambiguity and as people attempt to make sense of these ambiguities they are often able to choose preferred storylines and discourses. This can be seen in therapeutic settings when someone who may have told the story of the history of her abuse many times, having the effect on herself of then feeling like a victim, begins to recognize times of resistance and survival so that she gradually shifts into a storyline of survivor-hood and an identity of survivor. Stories are not all powerful, and through an exploration of the meaning-making process, a person is able to actively resist and make choices. White and Epston did not attempt to explain what element of a person was able to do this, although they did describe the need for a sense of community and support for people to be able to maintain their chosen changes.

I am not sure that Michael White and David Epston would have thought of the social construction of identity, the fluidity of identity through the possibility of moving from one storyline to another, and the ability to be agentive in this process as involving inconsistencies. Their focus was on practice, describing how to practice in a way that would not reinforce mainstream pathologizing discourses in therapeutic settings. In so much as they can be described as having developed a theory, it is a practice theory rather than a theory of the structure of the person, which is what they were standing up against much of the time due to the potentially normalizing power inherent with such structures.

White's Position on the Spiritual in Narrative Therapy

Before moving on to recent commentaries regarding narrative therapy, I will comment on White's position regarding spirituality. There is only one published interview where White (2000) answers questions about his thoughts on spirituality, which I have also presented in *The Narrative Practitioner* (Béres, 2014). He states he believes that there are primarily three ways of thinking about spirituality:

1 Ascendant, involving looking 'up' and 'out' to a possible Divinity as a guide to our lives
2 Immanent, involving looking inside or 'deep down', which he saw as possibly being more psychological in a manner as people attempted to live in accordance with their notion of their 'true nature'

3 Immanent/ascendant, involving a connection to one's inner soul as a way to become in touch with the ascendant Divine

He then goes on to say that, although he tends not to think about spirituality in any of these terms, what interests him is what he calls "spirituality of the surface", or what he suggests relates to material existence, and so with the "little sacraments of daily existence" (White, 2000, p. 145). He quotes an Australian novelist:

> [T]he little sacraments of daily existence, movements of the heart and invitations of the close but inexpressible grandeur and terror of things, [... are] the major part of what happens every day in the life of the planet and [have] been from the very beginning. To find words for that; to make glow with significance what is usually unseen, and unspoken to; that, when it occurs, is what binds us all, since it speaks immediately out of the centre of each of us; giving shape to what we too have experienced and did not till then have words for, though as soon as they are spoken we know them as our own.
>
> (Malouf in White, 2000, p. 145)

White goes on to highlight that he was particularly interested in the idea of 'little sacraments of daily existence', which are like Goffman's notion of 'unique outcomes', or events that have previously been overlooked or unstoried. He thinks these little events in people's lives can evoke a sense of the significant or of the sacred, which might be too easily overlooked since they are of the type that mainstream culture does not value. He does not refute Malouf's use of the term 'out of the centre of each of us' but does not necessarily support it either.

White has made comments in conference settings (e.g., 2005), suggesting ideas such as the 'inner self', or 'digging deep into the self', although 'beautiful ideas' influenced by certain cultural times and discourses, were not his focus. As a social worker and family therapist, he was focused on the daily events of life and the problems with living that people presented. He engaged with people from a position which highlighted and celebrated their possibilities in life. On the other hand, he worked in purposeful and thoughtful manners which respected Aboriginal culture and spirituality, and the Muslim culture and faith as they both struggled with discrimination in Australia. Although he would not have described himself as religious or spiritual, and some narrative therapists might argue that the language of the soul does not fit well within postmodern theories, I believe White would have been supportive of narrative practices developing in such a way as to respect people's spirituality and, therefore, also their descriptions of the soul. Indeed, I remember a fellow narrative-trainee, when I was initially visiting the Dulwich Centre for my first intensive learning block, described having previously attended a training event in her home country where

Michael White had been presenting his narrative ideas and how spiritual he had seemed to her. This did not strike me as particularly odd at the time, although I knew Michael would not have described himself as spiritual, necessarily. When I worked alongside Michael in an Indigenous community practice in Canada, I was aware of the true sense of interest and respect he showed for the Indigenous and non-Indigenous community members, which included a respect for their range of faiths and spiritualities. I also remember the last time I spoke with him in Australia, prior to his death the next spring, about his enthusiasm for having become involved with canvasing for the local Green Party. I remember him speaking of the harshness of the droughts with which Australia had been suffering, and I also recall what seemed like joy when a thunderstorm broke out in Canada and he went out onto the verandah of the Indigenous community agency in which we had been meeting to merely stand outside and breath in the cool damp air. For many, spirituality is linked to their experience of awe in nature and results in a need to care for the environment. In much the same way, I will be exploring in later chapters how the language of the soul does not require theorizing the soul as separate from the physical body, and rather can further contribute to a respect for the physical and all aspects of nature.

Recent Theoretical and Practical Developments in Narrative Therapy

Guilfoyle (2014) begins his post-structuralist account of the person in narrative therapy by suggesting there are two stances within narrative practices which he wonders how to reconcile: the power of discourses to socially construct identity and people's ability to resist that power. I agree that in his last book, *Maps of Narrative Practice* (2007b), White presents himself as a "therapeutic optimist" (Guilfoyle, 2014, p. 13), while also calling upon the "Foucauldian constitutionalist perspective" (p. 13). Although White touches on the impact of Foucault's contribution to his understanding of the history of the "habit of thought that constructs [...] internal understandings of people's lives" (White, 2007b, p. 25), he clarifies that in practice he is much more interested in "intentional state understandings versus internal state understandings" (White, 2007b, p. 100). In relation to a transcript of a therapeutic conversation included in the book, he says,

> These understandings of his actions were not referenced to any concept of an essential self, but instead provided an account of what he was actively and willfully engaging with and embracing in his acts of living. Rather than representing his actions as essences of his identity, these intentional understandings arrived at in these conversations were in harmony with particular themes of life to which [they] attributed overriding importance. It is these intentional understandings, and

> understandings that are centred on what people give value to, that are highly significant in rich storyline development.
>
> (White, 2007b, p. 101)

White continues to clarify what he means by internal versus intentional state understandings. He points out that examples of internal state understandings would be related to concepts such as the 'unconscious mind', humanist understandings of 'human nature', or even Western notions of the individualized 'self'. Influenced by Foucault, he is concerned that these have all contributed to a system of social control through 'normalizing judgments', which he believes replaced religion's control through 'moral judgments'. Intentional state understandings have to do with personal agency; He says people are able to live their lives according to their intentions, pursuing that to which they give value. He quotes Jerome Bruner's work on folk psychology to support his argument, saying all cultures have folk psychologies, which suggest how people "'tick,' what our own and other minds are like, [...] what are possible modes of life [...] and that the term was] [c]oined in derision by the new cognitive scientists for its hospitality toward such intentional states as beliefs, desire, and meaning" (Bruner in White, 2007b, p. 103). I argue that this shows how White was supportive of the notion of a person's 'mind', as well as the notion of socially constructed identities, and interested in how people's values and beliefs influence their choices in life. What concerned him was how certain types of ideas about the structure of a person would 'normalize' and attempt to control from an external position of power, while other ideas supported people's right to operate out of their own beliefs and values. Guilfoyle (2014), on the other hand, stresses that White is presenting inconsistencies within the Foucauldian framework of narrative therapy when he discusses peoples' ability to be active agents in their lives. Guilfoyle's (2014) answer to this is to return to Foucault and other post-structuralists to understand how resistance and agency can occur, but he continues to resist any possibility of an inner self, other than what might be socially constructed. This requires him to review Foucault's later work on ethics, which he also suggests presents inconsistencies.

Guilfoyle (2014) provides an interesting account of how as people resist a particular discourse, they might be engaged in positive resistance as they choose another discourse and storyline over the former. However, he also suggests that there are times when people engage in negative resistance as they merely say, 'No', to the dominant and problematic discourse without yet choosing or being informed by another. (This could be seen in the opening case example as Lydia had begun to stand up against her church's discourse, although she was not yet confident or sure what she wanted to choose in its place.) Although Guilfoyle recognizes that this happens in his clinical psychology practice with people, he argues that post-structuralist accounts regarding knowledge and power do not explain this. He then draws upon Foucault, Veyne, and Nietzsche who argue that every embodied individual operates like a center of energy that cannot be fully encapsulated by any one discourse. He says, "the body is not a singular, coherent physical object, possessing universal drives or needs, but 'a multiple phenomenon' composed of 'irreducible forces'" (Guilfoyle, 2014, p. 117). The body's multiplicity and complexity are what make it malleable and susceptible to the discourses which are more likely to offer the comfort of simplicity. This implies that a discourse provides order to the body's chaos, but in doing so "grants it what Fouacault [...] called a 'soul' – an enduring and deeply felt sense of one's self, in the form of a constituted subject – which becomes the 'prison of the body'" (Guilfoyle, 2014, p. 119). However, he moves on to say,

> We overflow our discursive imprisonment in the most banal and unintentional of ways: we cough, sneeze, laugh, or yawn when we're not supposed to; we stumble when we walk, or we move faster, more expansively, and take up more space than we should; we stammer and forget our lines, or we don't stick to the point – we use more words, tell stories, and speak louder than is expected. Our bodies groan under the weight of discourse and its restrictive, imprisoning disciplinary specification, and then we inevitably slip out from under it.
>
> (Guilfoyle, 2014, p. 121)

Ultimately, Guilfoyle chooses not to take either a strong social constructionist nor totally individualist approach, as he argues that a person "has capacity for personal agency insofar as his or her embodiment allows him or her to have effects in the world that are personally meaningful" (Guilfoyle, 2014, p. 132). In this way, Guilfoyle is able to sidestep the need to discuss the soul as anything other than a social construct, but his descriptions are helpful and remind us that the soul cannot be considered in isolation from the body and that our experiences of ourselves are constantly in flow and shifting across time, and not easily pinned down. This idea of the person in flow is a good reminder that people are always changing. Foucault's ideas and focus changed over time also, as did White's. They and their ideas perhaps contained ambiguities and inconsistencies but were also maybe merely evolving. As an example of this, I will discuss White's ideas about the 'absent but implicit', which he was developing and writing about at the time of his death.

The Absent but Implicit in Narrative Therapy

Four months before Michael White died, I attended a small advanced-training workshop (White, 2007a) which he offered at the Dulwich Centre. Eight of us spent a week with him particularly learning and practicing what he called 'an absent but implicit' conversation. He explained that he had not previously written about this, but he was beginning to think it was the most important of the conversational maps (guidelines) he had developed and he wished he had stressed it more. Following his death, his colleagues, Carey, Walther, and Russell, (2009) published an article about the "absent but implicit" as he had taught it to them, and I also presented a streamlined version of it in *The Narrative Practitioner* (2014).

Derrida's concept of différance particularly influenced White in relation to the practice of this type of conversation. Using Derrida's description of how a word ('a signifier') involves both a description of what it is attempting to represent ('the signified') and also its opposite, or what it is not, White became curious about what was implied people knew, but what was absent from their descriptions. For example, if someone complained about feeling hopeless White would not try to cheer them up or have them explore the emotion of hopelessness, but rather would assume that if someone used this word they would also have an idea of its opposite: at least the awareness of hope. If hopelessness was their normal way of being and they had never experienced hope in any manner they probably would not have complained about hopelessness. So, he would ask them questions to explore how they knew to not be satisfied with hopelessness and explore the history (the story) of how they knew something other than hopelessness. This approach assists people in becoming clearer about their preferences and values. In relation to Lydia again, whom I mentioned at the beginning of this chapter, in one session when she spoke about feeling let down by humanity because she felt her supervisor had been interacting inappropriately with many staff, and she was saddened to hear a friend had been terminated from her position, I asked her what her reactions to these situations were implying was of greatest importance to her. She went on to say that her valuing of relationships and social supports was what came to mind as underlying these concerns. She continued by describing how she had met with colleagues, and her friend, on two separate occasions since these concerning situations and this process of reaching out to others and supporting one another was at least a partial antidote to her feeling 'let down by humanity', and linked to her sense of spirituality, she said. Although space restrictions do not allow me to describe the absent but implicit conversation fully here, my aim in raising it is to highlight the manner in which White's ideas and practices were continuing to develop and how he had a curiosity about what was absent, but implied, in people's descriptions of their lives. Perhaps the soul could be described as another such element of a person's life that might often be absent from their descriptions of themselves, but also implied.

Experiences of the Soul in Narrative Therapy

Schwartz (1999) begins his chapter regarding the "release of the soul in psychotherapy" pointing out that he was led by his clients to the area of spirituality despite his own "nonreligious socialization and scientific training" (p. 223). As a family therapist influenced by systems theory, he explains that he was most often focused in his practice on parts of family systems but overtime the way people talked about their experiences made him begin to wonder who we are at the core. Saying that each family therapy model answers that differently, he also says, "[t]he most popular answer in family therapy now comes from the constructivist movement and informs the many versions of narrative therapy. This answer is that there is no core self" (Schwartz, 1999, p. 225).

Using a combination of a narrative therapy technique of externalizing and a structural family therapy technique of boundary-making, Schwartz provides an example of how he might ask a woman who was feeling extremely angry toward her son to attempt to separate herself from that angry part temporarily so that they could examine the anger and understand it better. He says that when he would ask people about that part of them left examining the externalized or boundaried element they would often answer, "That's not a part, that's my Self; that's my core or true Self; that's who I really am" (Schwartz, 1999, p. 226). He says he initially attempted to make sense of this through the lens of developmental psychology, thinking this was a sense of ego, but he did not understand how his clients who had suffered through childhoods with parents who had been negligent or abusive in their behaviours toward them could have internalized a good parent and developed a healthy ego. He goes on to say he had to deconstruct his assumptions and consider the possibility that this Self came from somewhere else. As his clients explored what they understood as their Self he began to hear of more experiences which he could only describe as spiritual. He goes on to say,

> I began to conceptualize the Self as the soul of the person – the place in them that was God, or through which God-like energy could flow. The more I read about the soul and how it was conceived by different cultures, the more this definition fit, and the more ironic it seemed that so many spiritual or religious traditions knew about and helped people access the soul while so few psychotherapies did.
>
> (Schwartz, 1999, p. 227)

For my purposes, I will not review the Internal Family Systems model which he suggests presents a way of working in which the Self and soul are synonymous. Rather, I want to reiterate his comment that social-constructionist approaches like narrative therapy have no way to theorize the place of the soul in their work, alongside his descriptions in practice of meeting with people who describe experiences of being very aware of their soul. He has gone on to develop a way of conducting therapy which he now sees as a spiritual experience but has not theorized how this notion of the soul fits within narrative practices, which is my aim. Despite this 'gap' regarding theorizing the soul, there are a handful of Christian counselors, spiritual directors, and pastoral counselors who have been writing about the use of narrative therapy in their professional practices.

Narrative Practices in Spiritual Direction and Pastoral Counseling

Neuger (2001) has written about a narrative pastoral approach to counseling women, describing how narrative practices are congruent with her feminist and womanist theology. She describes how narrative approaches can provide a method of engaging with women so that they can deconstruct the discourses which have had negative and controlling influence and then move to a position where they are empowered to give voice to their circumstances. She specifically describes these practices in relation to providing services to women who have experienced intimate partner violence, and depression, and those women who wish to gain greater clarity, make choices, build community, and manage the context of aging.

Cook and Alexander (2008) have edited a collection of essays in which they present conversations between Christian spirituality and narrative therapy. They admit some of the philosophical difficulties in bringing these two areas together, while also arguing for the effectiveness of narrative approaches for engaging in transformative work. Within this collection, McMenamin (2008) reflects upon "The Self God knows and the socially constructed identity". Although not using the language of the soul, his description of the Self that God knows shares commonalities with how some might describe soul, suggesting it is possible to live and work with the tensions offered by holding onto both the idea of a Self, or soul, and of a socially constructed identity.

Bidwell (2013) describes his religious identity as "Buddhist Christian" (p. 11) and his theological orientation as "Reformed and liberationist" (p. 11). He provides a narrative approach to the spiritual care of couples, also drawing upon understandings of the desert mothers and fathers. The ideas of the desert mothers and fathers "evolved in the third and sixth centuries among women and men hungry for God; they left the cities to practice a solitary, contemplative style of Christian spirituality in the deserts […] away from an emerging church hierarchy in the urban centers" (p. 32). Their contemplative practices which went on to influence monastic traditions and can be seen to be closely tied to the mystics' writings are fascinating and in the next chapter I will describe the links that I experience between Christian contemplative traditions, Buddhist mindfulness, and critical reflection. I believe the ongoing appeal of, and perhaps expanding interest in, the desert mothers and fathers has to do with their commitment to resisting the hierarchy of organized religion. As many people now describe themselves as spiritual but not religious, there appears to be a desire to connect to what provides a sense of meaning and purpose without being told what to think and how to behave by leaders in the church – often 'by white middle-aged men', as Lydia expressed in the opening case example in this chapter. Bidwell goes on to provide a practical approach to working with couples which also draws upon Gottman's extensive research on what makes or breaks relationships. I appreciate the breadth of ideas Bidwell is drawing upon in his book, and also continue to wish to explore more thoroughly the language of the soul, adding this language to the range of ideas which can influence clinical theory and practice.

Coyle (2014) describes and recognizes the power of stories and provides a clear and helpful description of how narrative therapy has assisted her in her practice of pastoral care. She describes how she had been yearning for a counseling approach that would honor "local stories, encourage the emergence of stories, and not hold a normative story as the standard for all stories" (p. 4) when she first was introduced to narrative therapy through a workshop offered by Jill Freedman and Gene Combs. She says that while seated in the workshop she whispered to a colleague that "this feels theological" (p. 4), which sounds similar to my colleague's impression of Michael White seeming 'spiritual'. Just as Neuger (2001) and Bidwell (2013) have done, Coyle also has identified how narrative therapy practices are congruent with, and supportive of, the social justice aims of liberation theology. However, she also suggests a limitation of Bidwell's work is that it provides a "rather sophisticated level of pastoral care skills pastors should possess in order to implement their proposed narrative practices" (p. 17). It appears to be her desire to keep descriptions of narrative practice skills simplified for students and pastors new to the field of counseling that results in her text in which she provides many concrete examples of how to engage narratively with congregations. It is a practical text which does not explore the language of the soul. I agree with Coyle, Neuger, and Bidwell that narrative practices are clearly consistent with liberation theology, as well as feminist and womanist theology, and appreciate their clear descriptions for people learning narrative practice skills within pastoral counseling fields.

In addition to the texts I have reviewed, Campbell (2020) recently facilitated a presentation for a North American Christian Social Workers (NACSW) training session in which she discussed her approach to responding to the effects of trauma in service users' lives. She described the influence of the sanctuary model of trauma-informed practice and how she pays attention to the effects of trauma on the body as she uses narrative therapy techniques and incorporates an interest in her clients' favorite spiritual narratives. She pointed out that for those of our service users who have an active Christian faith and practice, it may be useful to ask if there are any biblical stories that resonate for them in their journey of healing from the effects of trauma. She suggested this journey often involves three stages (like the three-act play of narrative practices, as presented in Duvall & Béres, 2011) where the first is focused on giving voice to the pain, the second is like a betwixt and between, or liminal, space, and the third involves reordering and movement into a preferred storyline. She pointed out that the biblical stories of the raising of Lazarus from the dead or the Easter story involving Jesus' death on Good Friday, waiting and grieving on Saturday, and the resurrection on Sunday might resonate for clients. However, she also pointed out the benefit of asking them if they could think of any biblical story that was most meaningful and significant for them in relation to their journey rather than the therapist suggesting one. In this way, she pointed out, therapists with no Christian faith or biblical knowledge can work with Christian clients of faith, who might appreciate this wholistic approach.

Campbell's idea of incorporating spiritual narratives in her narrative work was intriguing to me. Since I was working with Jane, who was wanting to talk about the effects of her experience of trauma and who also described herself as a devout fundamentalist Christian, I decided to inquire as to what biblical story might come to mind as resonating with some of her trauma story she had just shared. I was fascinated by her answer since it was not a story I ever would have thought of. I find this happens often in therapeutic discussions where those people consulting us are so creative and offer such fresh insights. Thankfully, narrative therapy's political and philosophical underpinnings propose a therapeutic position of "de-centered but influential" (White, 2007b) where we are not the expert of another's life and where we acknowledge the other person will always know their life and meaning-making patterns better than us. Jane laughed when I asked her about a biblical story that might resonate. She told me her favorite story was of the fall of the wall of Jericho in the Book of Joshua in the Old Testament, which she went on to describe: scouts from the Israelite army entered the city of Jericho where they met with Rahab, who agreed to help them, but they told her she would need to keep silent about their intentions and wait patiently, while also committing to spare her and her family from any harm when they captured the city. She assisted the scouts in leaving the city safely, and then waited as each day for seven days the Israelite army marched around the outer wall of the city blowing their trumpets. On the seventh day the wall of Jericho fell, the army entered the city, killing all but Rahab and her family. I was not at all sure of how this was similar in anyway to her own story, so I was curious and asked her if she could explain the links to me. She said it was due to how she had also felt silenced for so long in response to the trauma, and how it felt like she also had been going around in circles for some time. She said she felt she continued to be in that stage of the story in her own journey, but she also had great hope in the image of the walls falling and finally being freed. This image was one that she relied upon in later counseling sessions, also, as she looked back and could consider how her story was changing over time.

All of the authors and practitioners I have mentioned are contributing to the process of bridging the areas of spirituality and narrative practices, and I hope to also add to this area of theory and practice literature. However, none of them explore the language of the soul and the complexities and possibilities offered with this term, which is something I am interested in adding to the conversation.

Conclusion

In this chapter I have presented an account of the influences upon the development of narrative therapy in such a manner as to hopefully clarify its great contributions to the fields of family therapy and counseling, as well as to pastoral counseling, and spiritual direction. The fact that some of us have suggested there are inconsistencies, or gaps, within its theoretical base provides an opportunity to explore the literature on the soul in order to add to the ongoing and fluid discussions about the complexity of human existence.

As Tyler suggests in *The Pursuit of the Soul: Psychoanalysis, Soul-making and the Christian Tradition* (2016), "[t]he soul [...] is a linguistic signifier that allows us to gaze simultaneously at the physical and spiritual realms" (p. 181), requiring us to hold theology and psychology together, and calling for synthesis and creativity. As a pastoral theologian, psychotherapist, and spiritual director, he is well positioned to assist with the exploration of the various ways in which the soul has been conceptualized over thousands of years. Tyler's exploration of the soul is conducted with his particular psychoanalytic lens while I am bringing a narrative lens to this exploration, wishing to explore how the language of the soul might be woven into narrative theory and practice. Using an image that I particularly like, Tyler says, "the 'soul' is not some small furry beast lurking in the hinterland of ourselves but a linguistic signifier that is there to serve a performative function" (Tyler, 2016, p. 25). This is a useful image because it sits well with a narrative perspective that is committed to considering the power of language and discourses and how these have real effects in a performative manner in people's lives. Rather than thinking of the soul as a part of a person, like a 'thing', or located at some 'place' within a person, which we need to try and find and pin down, exploring the *language* of the soul offers an approach more consistent with the postmodern and social constructionist elements of narrative therapy.

Note

1 All names and identifying details of clients and case examples have been changed throughout this book.

References

Béres, L. (1999). Beauty and the beast: The romanticization of abuse in popular culture. *The European Journal of Cultural Studies*, *2*(2), 191–207.

Béres, L. (2002). Negotiating images: Popular culture, imagination and hope in clinical social work practice. *Affilia: Journal of Women and Social Work*, *17*(4), 429–447.

Béres, L. (2010). Narrative therapy ideas and practices for working with addictions. In R. Csiernik & W. S. Rowe (Eds). *Responding to the oppression of addiction: Canadian social work perspectives, 2nd Edition* (pp. 88–102). Canadian Scholars Press.

Béres, L. (2012). A thin place: Narratives of space and place, Celtic spirituality and meaning. *Journal of Religion and Spirituality in Social Work: Social Thought, 31*(4), 394–413.

Béres, L. (2013). Celtic spirituality and postmodern geography: Narratives of engagement with Place. *Journal for the Study of Spirituality, 2*(2), 170–185.

Béres, L. (2014). *The narrative practitioner.* Palgrave MacMillan.

Béres, L. (Ed.) (2016). *Practicing spirituality: Reflecting on meaning-making in personal and professional contexts.* Palgrave MacMillan.

Béres, L. (2017a). Narrative therapy ideas and practices for working with addictions. In R. Csiernik (Ed.). *Responding to the oppression of addiction: Canadian social work perspectives, 3rd Edition* (pp. 134–151). Canadian Scholars Press.

Béres, L. (2017b). Celtic Spirituality: Exploring the fascination across time and place. In B. Crisp (Ed.). *The Routledge handbook of religion, spirituality, and social work* (pp. 100–107). Routledge.

Béres, L. & Page Nichols, M. (2010). Narrative therapy group interventions with men who have used abusive behaviors: Are they any different? *Families in Society: The Journal of Contemporary Social Services, 91*(1), 60–66.

Bidwell, D. R. (2013). *Empowering couples: A narrative approach to spiritual care.* Fortress Press.

Blanton, P. G. (2005). Narrative family therapy and spiritual direction. *Journal of Psychology and Christianity, 24*(1), 68–79.

Campbell, C. (2020, July 27). Spiritual narratives in trauma work, *NACSW* webinar.

Canda, E. R. (1988). Spirituality, diversity, and social work practice. *Social Casework, 69*(4), 238–247.

Carey, M., Walther, S., & Russell, S. (2009). The absent but implicit: A map to support therapeutic inquiry. *Family Process, 48*(3), 319–331.

Cook, C., Powell, A., & Sims, A. (Eds). (2009). *Spirituality and psychiatry.* RCPsych Publications.

Cook, R. & Alexander, I. (Eds). (2008). *Interweavings: Conversations between narrative therapy and Christian faith.* CreateSpace Books.

Coyle, S. M. (2014). *Uncovering spiritual narratives: Using story in pastoral care and ministry.* Fortress Press.

Crisp, B. (2010). *Spirituality and social work.* Ashgate.

Duvall, J. & Béres, L. (2007). Movement of identities: A map for therapeutic conversations about trauma. In C. Brown & T. Augusta-Scott (Eds). *Narrative therapy: Making meaning, making lives* (pp. 229–250). Sage.

Duvall, J. & Béres, L. (2011). *Innovations in narrative therapy: Connecting practice, training and research.* W.W. Norton.

Guilfoyle, M. (2014). *The person in narrative therapy: A post-structuralist, Foucauldian account.* Palgrave Macmillan.

Hillman, J. (2007). *The soul's code: In search of character and calling.* Ballantine Books.

McMenamin, D. (2008). The self God knows and the socially constructed identity. In Cook & Alexander (Eds). *Interweavings: Conversations between narrative therapy and Christian faith* (pp. 143–162). CreateSpace Books.

Moore, T. (1992/2016). *Care of the soul: A guide for cultivating depth and sacredness in everyday life, 25th anniversary edition.* Harper Perennial.

Neuger, C. C. (2001). *Counseling women: A narrative, pastoral approach*. Fortress Press.

Peck, M. S. (2003). *The road less travelled: A new psychology of love, traditional values, and spiritual growth, 25th anniversary edition*. Touchstone.

Rogers, M. & Béres, L. (2017). How two practitioners conceptualise spiritually competent practice. In J. Wattis, S. Curan, & M. Rogers (Eds). *Spiritually competent practice in health care* (pp. 53–69). CRC Press.

Schwartz, R. C. (1999). Releasing the soul: Psychotherapy as a spiritual practice. In F. Walsh (Ed.), *Spiritual resources in family therapy* (pp. 223–239). The Guilford Press.

Tyler, P. (2016). *The pursuit of the soul: Psychoanalysis, soul-making and the Christian tradition*. Bloomsbury T & T Clark.

White, M. (1984). Pseudo-encopresis: From avalanche to victory, from vicious cycles to virtuous cycles. *Family Systems Medicine, 2*(2), 150–160.

White, M. (1995). *Re-authoring lives: Interviews and essays*. Dulwich Centre Publications.

White, M. (2000). *Reflections on narrative practices: Essays and interviews*. Dulwich Centre Publications.

White, M. (2005, April 11 & 12). Mapping Narrative Conversations. *Two-day training, sponsored by the Brief Therapy Training Centres International* (a division of Hincks-Dellcrest, Gail Appel Institute), Toronto, Ontario, Canada.

White, M. (2006, March 3). Addressing the Consequences of Trauma. *International Narrative Therapy Festive Conference*, Adelaide, SA, Australia.

White, M. (2007a, December 10–15). Level 2 Narrative Therapy Training. *Sponsored by the Dulwich Centre*, Adelaide, SA, Australia.

White, M. (2007b). *Maps of narrative practice*. W.W. Norton.

White, M. & Epston, D. (1990). *Narrative means to therapeutic ends*. W.W. Norton.

2 Critical Reflection and Contemplative Practices for Narrative Therapy

Laura Béres

When Morgan[1] telephoned the counseling agency where I work, she specifically asked to meet with a counselor who was comfortable with, and respectful of, her Pagan spirituality. She was referred to me since I am known within the organization as someone interested in making room for the topic of spirituality in counseling conversations and supportive of people's varying spiritual practices. Morgan's intake summary indicated that when she spoke on the phone to an intake worker she described the problem she wanted to address in counseling as her struggle with depression and anxiety. When Morgan and I first met, and after asking if she had any questions for me, I asked her what had been sustaining her during her experiences of depression and anxiety and she answered by describing her Pagan spiritual practices as aspects of her life which she found grounding. She also said her connections with others who shared her beliefs provided great comfort and a sense of community. One of the many rituals that she described as being important to her was her mindfulness and guided imagery practice that she said she used many mornings each week and which she identified as always improving those days in which she had taken the time to commit to the practice. I have also found that mindfulness and contemplative practices can be grounding, can assist me in being truly present to people I meet, support my critical reflection practice, and are one way in which I have been able to incorporate a respect for spirituality into my professional practice. Although people who consult with me in a counseling context may not think of mindfulness as being particularly religious or spiritual, both mindfulness and contemplative practices are supported by long and deep spiritual traditions. I will describe some of these traditions in this chapter since they have contributed to my approach to studying the language of the soul. This approach I have taken has also been influenced by the philosophical works of phenomenologists – particularly that of Edith Stein and Maurice Merleau-Ponty – which will be described in detail in later chapters.

Finlay states, "All phenomenologists agree on the need to study human beings in human terms. They therefore reject positivist, natural science methods in favor of a qualitative human science approach [… and] the

DOI: 10.4324/9781003137450-4

intertwining of science with art" (2009, p. 14). Indeed, particularly the study of human beings' experience of spirituality can benefit from an approach that is influenced by phenomenology with its openness to varying modes of examining any given experience. Finlay argues that "even Husserl's early work laid the foundations of the postmodern movement by highlighting varying modes of giveness and relativity of appearances. Here relativity of understanding is stressed instead of relativism as such" (p. 16). Having described a number of methodological approaches to studying practice phenomenologically, Finlay moves through the arguments about whether phenomenology is modern or postmodern, and then proposes that phenomenology "move forward and take its place beyond the modernist-postmodernist divide – the era some call post-postmodern" (p. 17). She quotes Denzin and Lincoln as saying phenomenologists will need to deal with this "new age where messy uncertain, multivoiced texts, cultural criticism, and new experimental works will become more common as well as more reflexive forms of fieldwork, analysis and intertextual representation" (Denzin & Lincoln in Finlay, 2009, p. 17). Although Denzin and Lincoln describe this as messy and uncertain, I would also suggest that taking various avenues for the study of a particular human experience can also add richness. In fact, my interest in exploring the language of the soul has come about partly due to critically reflecting upon my counseling practices with people, but also due to my own experiences with mindfulness and contemplative practices. So while I have immersed myself in the literature regarding the soul, and specifically the work of Teresa of Avila and Edith Stein, I have also continued to critically reflect upon my professional practices and to engage in contemplation, thus maintaining at least three different avenues toward gaining an understanding of the soul.

Having described narrative therapy in the previous chapter, I will begin this chapter by briefly exploring the manners in which critical reflection and narrative therapy share common foundational underpinnings and commitments, thereby demonstrating the manner in which critical reflection has offered a method of inquiry into my practice of narrative therapy; Critical reflection can be considered a methodology which may result in the development of theory in an inductive research manner. Through the critical reflection process it is possible to identify what could be described as a 'gap' between explicit espoused theories and the application and experience of those theories in practice. This process has contributed to my acknowledgment of what has felt missing in my practice as I explicitly commit to narrative therapy approaches, while realizing narrative therapy does not provide a theoretical framework for making sense of my experiences of how people discuss their souls. This is what I have experienced as the 'gap' in narrative therapy's theory which I described in the last chapter. Following this brief description of critical reflection, I will turn to a discussion of mindfulness and contemplative practices that have further enriched my critical reflection practice and my engagement with the work of the Christian mystics and philosophers which will be explored in later chapters. Specifically, I have been engaged in the following throughout this process: I have continued to maintain a narrative therapy practice and involvement in a critically reflective narrative consultation group; I have continued my contemplative and mindfulness practices individually and with the support of a spiritual director; I have also continued forms of reflective body work through my ongoing practice of Iyengar yoga, and walking each day; and I have immersed myself in the academic literature regarding the soul. The purpose of presenting descriptions of these various areas of inquiry and practice is to indicate the manner in which they are congruent with, and further enrich, one another, and also to be transparent regarding my positionality and the various paths I have taken to engage with this material. I have attempted to immerse myself in these concepts in an embodied and integrated manner rather than only through the intellect. I have not 'bracketed' my subjectivity and these personal experiences as some approaches to phenomenological research would suggest, but rather agree with those other researchers who suggest it is neither possible nor desirable to set aside our experiences and understandings in a research position; They suggest a critical self-awareness of our own subjectivity and interests is required, placing subjectivity in the foreground (Finlay, 2009). Finlay says, "Gadamer describes this process in terms of being open to the other while recognizing biases. According to him, knowledge in the human sciences always involves some self-knowledge" (Finlay, 2009, p. 12). This idea of self-knowledge will be further described while discussing mindfulness practices and the 'no-self' below.

The Relationship between Narrative Therapy and Critical Reflection on Practice

Both narrative therapy and critical reflection on practice are influenced by postmodernism, social constructionism, and critical theory perspectives alongside a commitment to social justice (Béres, Bowles, & Fook, 2011; Béres & Fook, 2020; Meidinger, 2020: White & Epston, 1990). These two practices developed separately from one another but have more recently begun to influence and inform each other. Critical reflection on practice as a particular approach to reflection has been described by its originator (Fook, 2002) as both a theory and a practice for examining events in a structured manner in order to uncover previously hidden assumptions and values with the purposes of developing and articulating new practice theories. More recently, we have described it in the following manner:

> Critical reflection involves learning from and making deeper meaning of experience through a process of unsettling and examining deeply hidden assumptions in order to create better guidelines for action and so improve professional practice and develop a more ethical and

> compassionate stance. It is informed by a reflexive awareness of how the whole self influences knowledge-making and behaviour by an appreciation of the link between language and power, an understanding of how personal experience is also social and political, and how individual beliefs can be changed in order to contribute to socially just change.
>
> (Béres & Fook, 2020, p. 3)

The process of critical reflection involves a person describing an incident from their practice (or from any aspect of life) upon which they have been ruminating. This description of the incident is often written and then shared with a small group of others who assist with stage one, which is like an exercise of deconstruction, in which the group members ask questions about the description of the incident through five theoretical frameworks, or lenses (Béres & Fook, 2020). The five theoretical frameworks are reflective practice; reflexivity; post-structural thinking and postmodern narrative practice; critical perspectives; and spirituality. Narrative practice and spirituality are new additions to the theory and practice of critical reflection, which previously has been described as containing four theoretical approaches: reflective practice, reflexivity, postmodernism and deconstruction, and critical social theory (Fook & Gardner, 2007). It is best if there is some time, at least one week, between stage one and stage two of the critical reflection process, to allow new thoughts or ongoing questions to settle or result in further ideas. Then the group reconvenes for stage two, asking the person who presented an incident to first describe where they have moved in their thinking about the incident and then asking questions again from the five theoretical frameworks, but this time with a more future-oriented approach that supports the person in considering how new insights and articulated values that were uncovered through stage one might be reconstructed and contribute to new commitments or future practices.

The critical reflection process has been clearly described in other places (Fook & Gardner, 2007; Béres & Fook, 2020), so I will not provide detailed descriptions here. My purpose in raising critical reflection is to highlight how it has provided me with a method of practice inquiry which aligns with narrative therapy practices and has proved to be a useful beginning step in the process of deconstructing and reconstructing experiences within narrative practices. However, in addition to critical reflection and narrative therapy sharing underlying theories, philosophical outlooks, and commitments to social justice, they both are able to open up the space for the consideration of spirituality and meaning-making. As I have suggested in the first chapter, narrative therapists take on a de-centered but influential therapeutic posture which ensures maintenance of a stance of curiosity regarding the life of the person who is consulting them. Although narrative therapists develop expertise in facilitating narrative conversations, therapists do not think of themselves as experts in diagnosis or in comparing the other's life to some external standard. Questions are asked in narrative conversations about what the other person's statements imply regarding their values, hopes, and preferences, and how they make meaning of their situations (Béres, 2014; Freedman & Coombs, 1996; White, 2007). In fact, being curious about the 'absent but implicit', and unique outcomes and preferred storylines provides simple openings to discussions about what keeps a person hopeful and what gives them a sense of meaning and purpose in life despite the situations which have brought them to counseling in the first place – similar to asking Morgan in the opening case example about what had been sustaining her. As I have experienced many times with people, this sense of meaning and purpose does not need to be related to organized religion and could just as easily be related to feeling connected to something greater when they are on a nature walk or drawing a sense of purpose and connection through their relationships. So, I, and others mentioned in the first chapter, have argued that the area of spirituality can be incorporated into narrative practices. This is based upon using a broad definition of spirituality: Canda (1988) defines it as "the human quest for personal meaning and mutually fulfilling relationships among people, the non-human environment, and, for some, God" (p. 243). Crisp (2010) suggests spirituality "provides the basis for us to establish our needs and desires for, understand our experiences of, and ask questions about, meaning, identity, connectedness, transformation, and transcendence" (p. 7). While there have been many of us arguing for the importance of including spirituality in counseling, social work, and narrative therapy practices, and while Gardner (2011) has previously written about "critical spirituality", the specific links between spirituality and critical reflection have only been articulated more thoroughly recently.

Fook (2017) has interestingly described how she was drawn to developing and practicing critical reflection over more than 20 years, and suggests that she has come, "somewhat shamefully I feel, to appreciate the role of spirituality in peoples' lives rather late in my own life and career" (p. 17). She suggests that having had the "good fortune to have very close friendships with people who both espoused and practiced a quiet yet substantial spirituality" (p. 17) and a life partner working in end-of-life care with whom she engaged in discussions about the bigger questions in life, have kept her "surrounded by the important questions which for many people their spirituality attempts to address" (p. 18). After years of being intrigued and excited by the process of critical reflection as she engaged in it herself and with colleagues, she indicates she realized that she had found greater meaning and purpose in life with critical reflection (p. 20). For Fook, this sense of meaning and purpose was also clearly connected to her commitment to social justice. Adding the fifth lens of spirituality to the four which had previously made up the critical reflection on practice model was in order to highlight the aspects of meaning-making and unearthing of personal values which are so much part of critical reflection (Béres & Fook, 2020; Fook, 2017). Indeed,

Fook and I have drawn upon Nussbaum's earlier work (1997) and her argument that reflection is in order to develop more ethical engagement with the world. In her later work, Nussbaum (2010/2016), drawing upon Socrates, also proposes that education not only prepares people for citizenship and employment, but also prepares them "for meaningful lives" (p. 9). She goes on to argue that this will require "cultivated capacities for critical thinking and reflection" (p. 10). Fook (2017) argues that the reason we learn from experience, and what education should be equipping us for, is to become more ethical, compassionate, and better citizens and members of the community.

Hunt (2016), reflecting on her own journey of reflective practice and her interest in spirituality over 20 years, draws upon Swinton's suggestion that defining spirituality runs the risk of making something immaterial a 'thing'. She explains Swinton would suggest it is more useful to focus on what spirituality does versus what it is: "in all its diverse forms, spirituality helps us pay a different kind of attention to the world" (Swinton in Hunt, 2016, p. 37). They both argue that this sort of attention assists us in focusing on crucial aspects of "being human and caring humanly" (p. 37). Although this links again to a commitment to social justice, she goes on to indicate this also can involve experiences of awe and wonder. However, what we pay attention to has significant implications and effects.

Hunt (2016) provides a description of how various orientations to reflective practice can be distinguished from one another based upon their main focus in the following few areas; Each reflective approach might consider education either domesticating or liberating, might focus more on people or systems, and then might have a more technical, deliberative, dialectic/critical, or transpersonal/spiritual orientation. On one end of the continuum the focus of reflection might be domesticating of students, focused on systems operating smoothly, and mostly interested in efficiency and effectiveness of practice. Still viewing education as more domesticating than liberating, a deliberative orientation focusing on individual people is more likely to support an individual's self-development within our current work systems and structures. Both the dialectical/traditional critical reflection and the transpersonal/spiritual orientations to reflective practice consider education as having the potential to be liberating. Hunt suggests the dialectic and Fook's original form of critical reflection have a focus more on systems than the person and would empower the individual but primarily with a focus on this leading to change in the work context. She argues that the transpersonal/spiritual orientation to reflective practice focuses more on people than systems and leads to what she calls "integration of individual's subjective/objective (inner/outer) experiences beyond the work environment" (2016, p. 44). I would add to her description that as the critical reflection model developed by Fook has incorporated a greater focus on spirituality it has begun to result in the possibility of both empowerment of the induvial so the individual can bring about change in the workplace and also this integration of inner and outer experiences. For me, this is experienced as a sense of congruence between the various aspects of my personal and professional lives. Hunt suggests this involves the practitioner asking the following types of questions: "How can I integrate my personal/ spiritual growth with my vocation? [and] What is my personal responsibility to myself and others?" (Hunt, 2016, p. 44). Certainly, as my journey over the past 30 years as a practitioner and 20 years as an academic has unfolded, my orientation to reflective practice has also shifted across these types of reflective practices. Although effective practice is still important, a focus on efficiency in order to limit waiting lists for service is not my main priority. My critical reflective practice, incorporating the transpersonal and spiritual, has led to my questions about how to make sense of and understand both my personal and my professional experiences; Many of us are attempting to understand and articulate how we can experience complex fluid identities as well as an ongoing coherent and ethical sense of the self along-side these fluid identities. As I have suggested earlier, I believe an exploration of the language of the soul will provide further ideas for how to consider these experiences.

Having explained how both narrative therapy and critical reflection are able to open up the space for the area of spirituality, I will now turn to a description of mindfulness and contemplative practices which can add further richness to the critical reflection process.

Contemplative Practices and Critical Reflection

Mindfulness

I first wrote about the links between mindfulness and reflective practice in a chapter for Hick's (2009) edited book, *Mindfulness and Social Work,* in which I also touched upon my beginning foray into considering the similarities between Buddhist mindfulness and Christian contemplative practices. Hick suggests, "[m]indfulness, with its emphasis on awareness of the present moment, is central to models of well-being within virtually all spiritual traditions" (p. 3), going on to say that it does not need to be connected to a particular religion or spiritual tradition and so is practiced in secular contexts such as social work and psychotherapy. Nonetheless, he highlights that the English term 'mindfulness' first appeared in translations of texts written in the Pali language approximately 2,600 years ago, which were texts inspired by Siddhartha Gautama, otherwise known as Buddha. He also suggests that the usage of the term has continued to evolve, and some forms of mindfulness practices incorporate meditation, particularly as they have been integrated into counseling practices such as acceptance and commitment therapy (ACT) and dialectical behavior therapy (DBT) (p. 3). He describes mindfulness as "purposefully paying attention to the present moment with an attitude of openness, nonjudgment, and acceptance" (p. 4).

Drawing upon Langer's formulation of mindfulness, Hick draws out her distinctions between mind*ful*ness and mind*less*ness. Whereas Langer describes mindfulness as consisting of "openness to novelty, alertness to distinction, sensitivity to differing contexts, implicit awareness of multiple perspectives, and an orientation to the present", mindlessness results in people not paying attention, and "relying rigidly on fixed categories [...] that limit their thinking and can lead to stereotyping and to mislabeling" (p. 6). Clearly, this practice and commitment to moving away from rigid categories and toward openness to learning from new experiences is consistent with, and can enrich, the theory and practice of critical reflection on practice and narrative therapy.

By describing mindfulness further as a practice of refocusing on 'being' rather than 'doing', Hick suggests human beings are often more like "human doings" not thinking at all, or, alternatively, lost in thoughts about the past or future and not fully aware of the present (p. 7). By being aware of the present moment it is possible to be aware of the "emergent nature of phenomena as they arise in consciousness [and...] the nature of attachments made to these phenomena as they arise" (p. 8). This is relevant to the work of phenomenologists which will be explored in more detail as I discuss the work of Edith Stein in chapter five. Interestingly, Hick also points out that some forms of mindfulness also incorporate body awareness, and I will explore Maurice Merleau-Ponty's incorporation of the body into the phenomenological approach in chapter six. However, of relevance to the role of critical reflection on practice, Hick then problematizes the manner in which research regarding spirituality has relied on positivist approaches, developing questionnaires for measuring different elements of mindfulness, rather than relying on phenomenological approaches and lived experience. Arguing that mindfulness is an embodied state of mind, he says that research in this area needs "to proceed from an embodied, open-ended, reflective mode" (p. 16).

With Hick's descriptions of mindfulness as a backdrop, I have explored how my understanding of reflective practice within my direct social work/therapeutic practice was enhanced by my beginning mindfulness practice and how, together, critical reflection and mindfulness provided me with a sense of the Buddhist notion of 'no-self', in contrast to the Western individualized and encapsulated sense of self (Béres, 2009). What I have been most interested in is how mindfulness and being fully present allows for greater awareness of thoughts, emotions, and bodily sensations which can then inform choices made about how to act in that moment, thereby improving our interactions with others in those moments, whether clients, students, friends, or family. Although mindfulness is sometimes taught to enhance self-care strategies, and also incorporated into some forms of therapeutic interventions, as mentioned above, my interest in mindfulness was regarding how it can assist me in being more attuned to what is going on in and around me, which leads to improved (ethical rather than efficient) practice. The approach to mindfulness which I have incorporated involves attempting to note and let go of thoughts, feelings, and sensations as they arise. This translates into practice in such a way that I can note which thoughts and sensations need to be 'let go of' (like those that might have to do with suddenly realizing I am hungry and wondering briefly what I might eat for dinner) and those which are pertinent and might inform my interactions in that moment (like a tingle which suggests that what was just said was of particular importance). Nonetheless, these experiences of noting and letting go of thoughts also led me to wonder about, as others have, what part of me is watching and letting go of those things, and whether there is anything else to me except those thoughts, feelings, and sensations.

Engler (2003) describes the nuances and complexities of these ideas of being aware of the self while also letting go of the self. He admits that early in his career he suggested, "You have to be a somebody before you can be a nobody" (p. 35), recognizing this idea was influenced by Western psychological developmental models. However, he moves on to argue that it is possible to both know oneself psychologically speaking while also letting go of that self in the practice of mindfulness more philosophically speaking. Although a psychoanalyst rather than a narrative therapist, Engler points out something that White (2007) has also highlighted from a Foucauldian point of view; the psychologically differentiated self is a fairly recent idea in the grand scheme of human history: it "is a product of the last three or four hundred years of Western civilization: an autonomous individual with a sense of differentiated selfhood having its own nuclear ambitions, goals, design, and destiny" (p. 50). Collectivist cultures are much more focused on a sense of self that is "embedded in a matrix of relations and as defined by those relations" (p. 51). From a postmodern, or maybe even post-postmodern, perspective, I am interested in these different ideas about the self. There is no need to set up a binary and certainly no need to choose which is correct since they can both be experienced. In fact, Engler goes on to review four different ways of experiencing the self. The first description of an experience of self is as multiple and fluid as we are able to see ourselves being different in different contexts. The second is as much more integral and constant, as there continues to be a sense of 'myself' across various situations in which I might present differently. The third he describes as 'unselfconscious' which is more usually experienced in meditative and mystical experiences, when there is full and heightened awareness at the same time as there is a feeling of losing oneself in the wonder of that moment (for instance, while looking at a beautiful sunset). Engler suggests this third sense of self might also be experienced in a therapeutic context when the therapist is fully engaged in the therapeutic process. However, it is the fourth sense of self that is more like the notion of Buddhist 'no-self' which does not fit comfortably within Western psychological frameworks. He describes this experience by initially drawing upon Freud's observation that the ego can make itself an object of its own observation, but that we cannot observe our observing self, saying "detaching our 'self' from awareness in order to observe it is impossible because we *are* that awareness" (p. 66). He says,

> I witness the process of thinking, feeling, sensing, and perceiving as a series of discrete and discontinuous events, each arising and passing away without remainder. In this experience of complete discontinuous change, a Copernican revolution occurs. 'Things' disappear. What is apparent is only events on the order of milliseconds. Not only is everything changing all the time, there are no 'things' that change. Any notion of an enduring inherent self, a solid body, a durable perceptual object, even a fixed point of observation like an 'observing self' becomes completely untenable.
>
> (Engler, 2003, p. 69)

Although each of us can have a sense of an enduring feeling of 'myself' we can also have this experience of feeling as if things, ideas, and even 'self' only exist in relation to other things. This type of experience of 'self' sits relatively comfortably with narrative ideas about the social construction of identities and the externalizing of problems.

Bidwell (2018) offers some interesting explorations regarding the lives of spiritually fluid people which are helpful here, especially since he has also written about narrative approaches to spiritual care (2013), and his descriptions of the fluidity of spiritual identity resonate with underlying theories of narrative practices. He points out that stating his identity is both a Buddhist and a Christian might seem rather ironic since both faith traditions dispute that we can claim an identity for ourselves. While Christian doctrine would suggest Christian identity comes from, or is celebrated through, baptism, Buddhists reject the concept of identity; "the doctrine of no-self (anatta) instead affirms that nothing – not people, not flowers, not animals, not houses, not nations – has an inherent self or identity" (p. 77). However, much like Engler, he also recognizes that this ephemeral state is not how we experience our day to day identities. He goes on to ask,

> If we need identities to be fully human and to live well with others, then how do we make sense of these religious truths? What would it mean to live as if identity doesn't really exist and/or comes from somewhere beyond us? It's helpful, from my perspective, to see identity as a collection of meanings, negotiated with others. My identity doesn't come from inside me but emerges *between* me and others during shared experiences like washing dishes, following traffic laws, honoring parents, celebrating birthdays [...].
>
> (Bidwell, 2018, pp. 77–78)

Bidwell's exploration of the lives of spiritually fluid people is fascinating, as he highlights the microaggressions spiritually fluid people experience as, for example, they are asked to identify as belonging to one religion, another, or none on a hospital intake form, thus feeling their complex beliefs are minimized or ignored. He describes how some spiritually fluid people may be born into multifaith families while others might choose to move from one faith tradition to another and then later incorporate both. Most people who "choose multiplicity begin by emphasizing the similarities between traditions; only later do contradictions become important" (p. 47). This process begins with assimilating new traditions into past traditions and then as the nuances of the two traditions are more fully understood accommodations are made to existing religious ideas. Bidwell argues, few spiritually fluid people could be described as appropriating or exploiting traditions but are rather borrowing from other traditions or recognizing the complexities of influences across traditions. For instance, he explains,

> Prayer beads – commonly known as rosaries – were original to Buddhism, transmitted to Islam, then adopted by Christians during the Crusades. Christians adopted and adapted Jewish texts. Muslims bow in prayer in part because Jews did, and Jews stopped bowing in prayer to distinguish themselves from other Abrahamic faiths. As Buddhism, initially a reform of Hindu thought and practice, moved east into China, Japan and Korea and north into Tibet, it incorporated Confucian, Taoist, and Bon philosophies and senses of spirituality. Thomas Merton's description of *le point vierge*, the still, small spark at the center of humans that belongs entirely to God, has inspired Christians for decades – but the Catholic monk and mystic borrowed the idea from a medieval Muslim mystic without identifying the sourse.
>
> (Bidwell, 2018, p. 28)

I find these descriptions interesting as I look back to the chapter I wrote over ten years ago now about mindfulness and reflective practice. Perhaps I was in an assimilating phase as I was wondering about the ways in which Christian centering prayer might be like mindfulness. Indeed, Bourgeault (2004) describes the process and results of centering prayer in a similar manner to the above description of mindfulness leading to an experience of 'no-self', as we recognize that fears and self-talk are merely thoughts of which we are able to let go. In that earlier chapter, I also quote a favorite passage from Merton:

> I wind experiences around myself and cover myself with pleasures and glory like bandages in order to make myself perceptible to myself and to the world, as if I were an invisible body that could only become visible when something covered its surface.
>
> (Merton, 2003, p. 37)

In this way, Merton seems to be problematizing this common reliance on the external 'stuff' of life and so suggesting we attempt to separate or detach ourselves from these experiences which we wind about ourselves. He says we should also try to detach ourselves from our preconceived notions of what might provide pleasure, even from the wish to experience mindfulness or prayer in a particular peaceful or pleasurable manner; The more we are attached to wanting the experience to be a certain way the more we are apt to be disappointed and close ourselves down from the opportunity to experience something unexpected. Now, looking back I see in Merton's writing some of what Bidwell has proposed about the potential influence of a medieval Muslim mystic, and I also see similarities to the Celtic and medieval Christian mystics. Merton's description will resonate when I explore Teresa of Avila's description of the Interior Castle in chapter four, and Edith Stein's descriptions of the layers of the person in chapter five.

Christian Contemplative Practices

Keating has stated that he believes the rush by people in the West to the Eastern practices of mindfulness is a symptom of a spiritual hunger and indicative of what is lacking in the West (Keating, 2003, p. 31). He goes on,

> I have also noticed that those who have been on an Eastern journey feel that much more comfortable about the Christian religion when they hear that a tradition of contemplative prayer exists. Centering prayer as a preparation for contemplative prayer is not something that someone invented in our day. Rather it is a means of regaining the traditional teaching on contemplative prayer and of making this teaching better known and more available. The only thing that is new is trying to communicate it in a methodical way. One needs help to get into it and follow-up to sustain and grow in it.
>
> (Keating, 2003, p. 31)

It was on first reading this statement that I was motivated to turn back to my own Christian traditions to learn about these contemplative practices, partly because I had been worried that it could seem as though I was appropriating Buddhist traditions (I had not read Bidwell's reassurances to the contrary at that point), and partly due to a curiosity regarding the story of how these more spiritual and mystical traditions within Christianity had been downplayed or assumed to be only available to spiritual leaders. Religious studies scholars and theologians will be familiar with this history, but it was only through my growing interest in whether there was a history of Christian contemplation that was similar to Buddhist forms of mindfulness that I also learned about the desert fathers and mothers (versus the Church fathers) and the rich contemplative practices that have been passed down through the monastic tradition.

Bourgeault describes the Christian faith as being conveyed over time through "three streams: Scripture, Doctrine, and Tradition" (2004, p. 58). She goes on to suggest the strongest influence on centering prayer runs through tradition: from the desert mothers and fathers in the 3rd to 6th centuries and on through the Benedictine monastic tradition. Although she argues that it is through the stream of tradition that contemplative prayer and, much more recently, centering prayer have been passed on and developed, she does also point out that some Christian scholars have examined scriptural accounts of Jesus' prayer for guidance as to how to practice contemplative prayer. She says that we can assume Jesus was a contemplative, which she describes as involving "the intentional alteration between contemplation and action [as] one of the fundamental rhythms of his being" (p. 59). She points to his withdrawal into the wilderness after his baptism, his withdrawal to far shores of Lake Galilee before the miracle of the loaves and fishes, and to the garden of Gethsemane prior to his crucifixion. She says, "his pattern was to withdraw into solitude to listen more deeply to the word of God and unite his being to the divine Will" (p. 59). At this point she does admit it is not possible to know whether Jesus was engaged in cataphatic (sometimes spelled, 'kataphatic') or apophatic prayer; cataphatic prayer is probably what most people in formal religious traditions think of as prayer: "it engages our reason, memory, imagination, feelings, and will" (p. 31). In this form of prayer, we might speak (aloud or silently) the words of prayers we learned as children, or we might follow along in books as prayers are read aloud in a religious service. We might ask or thank God for something as we speak, rather than attempt to listen to God. The apophatic form of prayer does not use reason, imagination, or the other faculties engaged in cataphatic prayer, and is often described as formless or as the "*via negativa* ('the way of negation')" (p. 32). Apophatic prayer still requires a subtle use of the faculties, and Bourgaeult suggests these faculties are the spiritual senses which are more often ignored as we are so much more aware of the everyday senses upon which we usually rely. She describes us as living normally in a state of ordinary awareness, but that it is possible to develop a deeper level of spiritual awareness and divine awareness; she represents these forms of awareness in concentric circles with divine awareness being in the inner circle (p. 8). Bourgeault shows how accounts of how Jesus described payer in John's and Mathew's gospels influenced John Cassian's teaching about contemplative prayer in the 5th century. In particular, his use of Jesus' metaphor of "in secret" when describing how to pray was "a recognized category in Near Eastern traditions. In later Sufi texts (which built on the spiritual foundation of Syriac Christianity, the most immediate repository of Jesus' own lived tradition and teaching), the term refers specifically to prayer that is hidden from the outer faculties" (p. 60). She also says this idea of going to your room and closing your door to pray in secret would correspond to what the desert mothers and fathers would have called entering that "cave of your heart" (p. 60), where divine awareness and listening to God is more possible.

Although Christianity began as a small and marginalized belief system with its followers regularly persecuted, the Christian Church had become an imperial religion in the early 4th century. For some, the power and status involved with this new position were not consistent with their beliefs about how to authentically practice their faith (perhaps in a similar manner to how some today would prefer to identify as spiritual rather than be part of a religious organization). These were the people who turned to the Egyptian and Syrian deserts for a more solitary and simple life. "Their teachings and practices furnish the curriculum of Christianity's first and in some ways still most influential school of inner awakening" (Bourgeault, 2004, p. 61). In the 1960s Merton began to write about the influence of the wisdom of the desert mothers and fathers, suggesting their grounded spirituality was like that of the Zen masters, as they suggested a life of praying without ceasing in everything that is being done, mindfully engaging in whatever activity is being pursued. However, Bourgeault again cautions that we cannot be sure the desert mothers and fathers were actually teaching apophatic as well as cataphatic forms of prayer since they did rely on the psalms, much like centering prayer relies on a word or mantra, to focus and return the mind if it began to wander. Nonetheless, she concludes that "[t]he stepping from cataphatic into apophatic perception simply by stilling the faculties is such an innate soul wisdom that it's hard to believe it would remain unknown in a spiritual crucible as intense as that first great desert proving ground" (p. 65). Bourgeault then proceeds to describe how the Christian contemplative traditions were maintained within Benedictine monasteries, and how it was therefore not surprising that the more recent restorers of these traditions, Merton, Keating, and Main were all Benedictine monks, or influenced by this tradition, themselves.

The descriptions of how to live a Benedictine monastic lifestyle are primarily to be found within the 6th century *Rule of St. Benedict*, which has been described more recently in terms of how it can be incorporated into modern daily life outside of a monastery. However, Stewart (1998) points out that monastic life had already become well-established by the time Benedict became a monk; "[I]nformal ascetical communities, often home-based, had long been part of the Christian landscape in places as far apart as Rome, Asia Minor and Syria" (p. 17). In fact, the ascetical life of the 4th-century desert mothers and fathers influenced the monasteries but, despite the ongoing commitment to an ascetical life, as the monasteries spread through Italy, Gaul, and North Africa, bishops within the Church hierarchy and outside of the monasteries began to pressure them for greater regulation and structure of their life (Stewart, 1998). This resulted in *Rules*, like the *Rule of St. Benedict*, being developed.

Prior to any involvement in the monasteries, Benedict had spent time as a hermit in a cave near modern-day Subiaco in Italy, which is where he was found by nearby monks, and, recognizing his holiness, they asked him to become their spiritual leader. Stewart (1998) describes the resulting ups and downs of Benedict's involvement with setting up various monasteries, including an attempted poisoning of him by the monks who had asked him to be their spiritual leader. Benedict returned to living in solitude from time to time, and then in approximately 530 CE went to the mountain of Casinum where he razed the temple of Apollo and built two oratories for preaching (Stewart, 1998, p. 25), thus founding what has become known as Montecassino. The abbey has been severely damaged and rebuilt several times since then (abbaziamontecassino.org/abbey/en). However, the period in the 6th century in which he was founding this new monastic community would have been a time and context that would have required Benedict to focus on the need for balance and moderation in his *Rule*. Taylor argues that many monks in Benedict's day would have looked to the examples of the early Egyptian desert monks as a type of monastic hero. He says,

> As romantic as all this sounds, the European monks failed to live up to the tradition of the desert monks. Instead, they went to the opposite extreme, living lives of undisciplined license. Into this atmosphere, Benedict introduced his humane approach of zealous moderation, ordinariness, and balance.
>
> (Taylor, 1989, p. 32)

Benedict's focus on the benefits of balance and order (rhythm) for a healthy life has been described as one of his most significant discoveries and most useful pieces of advice. This balance ensures space and time for labor, sleep, and study as well as for leisure and contemplation, which people can too easily discount in the busyness of contemporary society (Pieper, 2009). Taylor (1989) and Chittister (2004) explain the flexibility present within Benedict's *Rule*, since he provides suggestions for how to live a balanced life but also often adds that these suggestions can be adapted if necessary. The *Rule*, therefore, is not a rigid legislation with laws to be adhered to, and the only thing like a vow that a monk is asked to make is to commit to a life of "stability, *conversatio*, and obedience" (Taylor, 1989, p. 15). Taylor explains that *conversatio* is not usually translated into English since no English word can capture all the nuances of the term. Stability is related to commitment to the community within the monastery, but outside of the monastery could be considered a commitment to the relationships in our own lives. *Conversatio* provides a sense of movement within that stability, since it involves a commitment to continually return to the spiritual journey we have undertaken. This recognizes that whatever our initial plans are for committing to a particular way of life we will often become distracted and can benefit from turning back. Obedience, Taylor suggests, was particularly needed in the chaotic times in which the *Rule* was first written, but also represents a Christian commitment to attempting to discern and follow God's will, rather than primarily putting our own wants first.

Within Benedict's *Rule* was also the suggestion that life be made up of a balance of prayer, study, and work (which originally would have most usually been a physical form of labor) (Taylor, 1989). Pratt and Homan (2000) describe people following Benedict's rule as "delightfully sensible people living simple and balanced lives. They find the time for play as well as prayer" (2000, p. 113). They say Benedict understood a need for balance, suggesting there must be time for everything: "Work. Sleep. Food. Companionship. Solitude. Noise. Silence. Reading" (p. 162), arguing people can become burned out on the one hand, or self-absorbed on the other, with too much of one or another of these elements in their lives. Pratt and Homan (2000) also suggest that these delightfully sensible people have a joy for life since this balanced approach to life also involves time for fun (p. 114). Indeed, Patrick Moore, in private communication, has highlighted that it is useful to consider the origins of the word "school" when we think of the proposition to be committed to "prayer, study, and work". Moore has pointed out that the Latin word "*schola*" is usually translated as "school" but carries within it more than the English word suggests today. *Schola* implied a break from physical labor/work and a time for ease and leisure in order to be able to learn and be part of learned conversations. Alongside all of this is also commitment to simplicity and frugality, which suggests a detachment from "things" and a focus on others' needs as well as our own (Taylor, 1989, p. 63).

I have spent some time discussing Benedictine spirituality as it was suggested it should be incorporated in the whole of life rather than focusing only on Benedictine forms of contemplation, since I believe the two are intrinsically linked and inform one another. A Benedictine life was not only made up of prayer, but prayer was to form just as an important part of a person's life as physical labor/work and study/leisure, with each part of that balanced life informing the others. However, returning to the topic of prayer, the greatest legacy from the Benedictine approach to prayer is the practice of "*lectio divina*; and specifically, [...] the fourth stage of *lectio*, known as *contemplatio*, or contemplation" (Bourgeault, 2004, p. 65). Bourgeault describes the four steps as contributing to the movement from cataphatic forms to apophatic forms of prayer, relying less and less on the intellect and an opening to just being in silence. The first step of this practice is *lectio*, or reading, where a short verse of scripture is read. The second step is *meditatio*, or meditation upon what was read and the associated thoughts and feelings. The third step is *oratio*, or a cataphatic form of prayer where thoughts are put into words and spoken to God. The fourth is *contemplatio*, or contemplation, where "all the mental and even emotional work is suspended. The faculties are stilled, and one simply rests in the presence of the divine" (Bourgeault, 2004, p. 67). Bourgeault goes on to say,

> It is exactly here, at this 'still point of the turning world,' that the Benedictine monks intuitively recognized the true home of meditation

> within Christian spiritual tradition, and also its authentic context. Unlike the positioning of meditation in Eastern spiritual traditions, as a spiritual practice in and of itself [...] it is not an isolated activity, to be undertaken too far removed from the Word. [...] *Contemplatio*, becomes a "womb", in a sense, in which scripture is enfolded in stillness and then reborn, deep within a person's heart, in a quickened conscience and more vibrant archetypal imagination.
>
> (Bourgeault, 2004, p. 67)

So, despite the similarities between Eastern forms of mindfulness practices, Bourgeault is attempting to point out that as the more recent form of centering prayer was developed as a derivative of contemplative practices it was not attempting to copy an Eastern method but rather refresh a branch of the Christian tradition. Centering prayer was to provide a method for people to experience the fourth step of *lectio divina*, *conetmplatio*, "where the faculties are left behind and one simply enters stillness" (p. 68).

Conclusion

In presenting these detailed descriptions of critical reflection on practice and the history and tradition of Christian contemplative practices I have hoped to provide some context for counselors without a background in Religious Studies or Theology. I have pointed out some similarities and differences between Eastern forms of mindfulness and Western Christian contemplative practices, showing the influence of Buddhist traditions and Eastern Christian desert traditions on current day contemplative practices. In this way, I have highlighted that I have been most interested in the study of spirituality and contemplative practices as they have been passed down through tradition from the desert mothers and fathers and through the Benedictine monasteries to today. These contemplative practices are influenced by the need for balance and commitment to stepping back from the busyness of the world but then also stepping back into the world and working for social justice. Whenever I argue for the need to make space for the area of spirituality in counseling practices and critical reflection I always stress that this is to honor the other's values and sense of meaning and purpose and not in order to proselytize or teach doctrine. Bourgeault's description of Christian beliefs and practices being passed down through scripture, doctrine, and tradition helps clarify these distinctions and offers the opportunity for me to stress my interest is particularly in regards to what has been passed down through tradition. As I have pursued an exploration of the language of the soul, I have been most drawn to those writers who also could be described as being part of the tradition passed on from the desert mothers and fathers through the monasteries. This will be particularly evident in the descriptions of Teresa of Avila's work in the 16th century.

Finally, I have also presented these descriptions of contemplative practices since they offer an approach for enriching critical reflection practices and have provided one of the avenues through which I have engaged with my own experience of spirituality while I have read others' descriptions of the language of the soul.

Note

1 All names and identifying details of clients and case examples have been changed throughout this book.

References

Béres, L. (2009). Mindfulness and reflexivity: The no-self and the reflexive practitioner. In S. F. Hick (Ed.). *Mindfulness and social work* (pp. 57–75). Lyceum Books.

Béres, L. (2014). *The narrative practitioner*. Palgrave MacMillan.

Béres, L., Bowles, K., & Fook, J. (2011). Narrative therapy and critical reflection on practice: A conversation with Jan Fook. *Journal of Systemic Therapies, 30*(2), 8–97. Doi: 10.1521/jst.2011.30.2.81

Béres, L. & Fook, J. (Eds). (2020). *Learning critical reflection: Experiences of the Transformative learning process*. Routledge.

Bidwell, D. R. (2013). *Empowering couples: A narrative approach to spiritual care*. Fortress Press.

Bidwell, D. R. (2018) *When one religion is not enough: The lives of spiritually fluid people*. Beacon Press.

Bourgeault, C. (2004). *Centering prayer and inner awakening*. Cowley Publications.

Canda, E. R. (1988). Spirituality, diversity, and social work practice. *Social Casework, 69*(4), 238–247.

Chittister, J. (2004). *The Rule of St. Benedict: Insight for the ages*. Crossroad Publishing.

Crisp, B. (2010). *Spirituality and social work*. Ashgate.

Engler, J. (2003). Being somebody and being nobody: A reexamination of the understanding of self in psychoanalysis and Buddhism. In J. D. Safran (Ed.). *Psychoanalysis and Buddhism: An unfolding dialogue* (pp. 35–79). Wisdom.

Finlay, L. (2009). Debating phenomenological research methods. *Phenomenology and Practice, 3*(1), 6–25.

Fook, J. (2002). *Social work: Critical theory and practice*. Sage.

Fook, J. (2017). Finding fundamental meaning through critical reflection. In L. Béres (Ed.). *Practising spirituality: Reflections on meaning-making in personal and professional lives* (pp. 17–29). Palgrave.

Fook, J. & Gardner, F. (2007). *Practicing critical reflection: A resource handbook*. Open University Press.

Freedman, J. & Coombs, G. (1996). *Narrative therapy: The social construction of preferred identities*. W.W. Norton.

Gardner, F. (2011). *Critical spirituality: A holistic approach to contemporary practice*. Ashgate.

Hick, S. F. (Ed.) (2009). *Mindfulness and Social Work*. Lyceum.

Hunt, C. (2016). Spiritual creatures? Exploring an interface between critical reflective practice and spirituality. In Fook, J., Collington, V., Ross, F., Ruch, G., & West, L. (Eds). *Researching critical reflection: Multidisciplinary perspectives*. (pp. 34–47). Routledge.

Keating, T. (2003). *Open mind, open heart: The contemplative dimension of the gospel.* Continuum.

Meidinger, N. (2020). Finding exception: Application of narrative practice in professional critical reflection on practice. In L. Béres & J. Fook (Eds). *Learning critical reflection: Experiences of the Transformative learning process* (pp. 44–54). Routledge.

Merton, T. (2003). *New seeds of contemplation.* Shambhala. (Original work published 1961.)

Nussbaum, M. C. (1997). *Cultivating humanity: A classical defense of reform in liberal education.* Harvard University Press.

Nussbaum, M. C. (2010/2016). *Not for profit: Why democracy needs the humanities.* Princeton University Press.

Pieper, J. (2009). *Leisure: The basis of culture.* Ignatius Press. (Original work published 1952.)

Pratt, L. C. & Homan OSB, D. (2000). *Benedict's way: An ancient monk's insight for a balanced life.* Loyola Press.

Stewart OSB, C. (1998) *Prayer and community: the Benedictine tradition.* Darton, Longman and Todd Ltd.

Taylor, B. C. (1989). *Spirituality for everyday living: An adaptation of the rule of St. Benedict.* The Liturgical Press.

White, M. (2007). *Maps of narrative practice.* W.W. Norton.

White, M. & Epston, D. (1990). *Narrative means to therapeutic ends.* W.W. Norton.

Part II
The Language of the Soul

3 A Timeline for the Language of the Soul, from Plato to Current Day

Laura Béres

As I was recently leaving a hospital parking garage, I overheard a woman at the payment kiosk say, 'I owe my soul to this parking garage', and her use of 'soul' jumped out as an interesting example of one of the many ways 'soul' is used in conversation. From the postmodern position of a narrative psychotherapist, I am curious not only in how any particular word, such as 'soul', is defined and understood today but also in the discourses it calls upon and the traces of older traditions which can be found within it. Within a therapeutic context, when Lydia, whom I mentioned in the first chapter, said it was important to her to 'feed her soul', I asked her about what that meant to her, and she suggested it was hard to put into words, although at the same time it was also very much a 'taken-for-granted' concept for her.

Moore (2016) argues anyone interested in understanding psychology, psychiatry, or psychotherapy, which all rely on the Greek word for soul (*psyche*), should restore the original sense of soul by making connections between psychology and spirituality (p. XIII). He goes further by contending that reading literature and poetry will assist with this project, and, as someone living in New England, he particularly suggests the poetry of Ralph Waldo Emerson, Emily Dickinson, and Walt Whitman, in whose work the word 'soul' is often found (p. XIII). For example, one of *my* favorite poems of Emily Dickinson's begins, "Hope is the thing with feathers, That perches in the soul, And sings the tune without the words, And never stops at all" (http://www.public-domain-poetry.com/emily-elizabeth-dickinson/hope-13626). I sometimes share this poem with students and discuss the need to support hope, which Dickson suggests perches in the soul, and which can seem fragile at times for those people who consult us in therapeutic contexts.

This return to the humanities alongside the study of spirituality and the soul is one response to what Tyler (2016) describes as a time of crisis for psychology. He quotes Slater as saying,

> Materialism and numbers have eclipsed interiority. Cognitive-behaviourism and neuroscience dominate the landscape – flatlands where subjects are quantified, therapies are determined economically, and pills

DOI: 10.4324/9781003137450-6

> are given before anyone asks, 'what's wrong?' [...] Psychology has placed itself inside a Skinner box – a place with an empty interior where psychologists map the brain and observe activity.
>
> (Slater in Tyler, 2016, p. 9)

Although narrative therapy has not historically been interested in the language of the soul, it has also raised concerns about limiting people through a scientific-rational lens to their cognitions, behaviors, and neuroscientific observations. As pointed out in chapter one, narrative therapy has been interested in supporting people's agency, intentions, values and preferences, and curious about "the little sacraments of daily existence, movements of the heart and invitations of the close but inexpressible grandeur and terror of things, that are the major part of what happens every day in the life of the planet" (Malouf [a novelist and poet] in White, 2000, p. 145). As White has suggested, these little events in people's lives can evoke a sense of the significant, or of the sacred, which might be too easily overlooked since they are of the type that mainstream culture does not value, and much of psychology and psychotherapy has overlooked.

In this chapter, since I am introducing the language of the soul to narrative therapy, I will review some of the various ways in which the soul has been described over the past 2,500 years so as to trace how these ideas have shaped particular ways of thinking about the soul within a Western tradition. These ideas were circulating prior to the development of the Christian tradition, and have been influenced by Hindu, Buddhist, and Indigenous traditions. Given my own particular cultural location and heritage, I will be focusing on how the language of the soul has developed within a Western context that is primarily Christian, although more secular or 'spiritual but not religious' in recent times. I hope that those people within other cultural and spiritual traditions will take up this project and write about how the soul is described within their religious and geographical contexts. At times it feels as though it would take many lifetimes to have the time to study and understand all the various faith traditions in the detail necessary to describe how the soul is understood in each and every one of them with the care this would deserve. However, despite many people's distrust of organized religion, as touched upon in the last chapter, there nonetheless continues to be an interest in spirituality and the care of the soul today.

To begin this exploration of the language of the soul, Tyler presents a helpful etymological note:

> The English *soul,* like the German *Seele,* has roots in the Gothic *saiwala* and Old German *saiwalô,* which for Jung can be linked with the Greek Αῖολος/*aiolos*: mobile, coloured, iridescent [...], also the mythical keeper of the Winds. Other commentators [...] link it to the Proto-Germanic, *saiwaz,* literally 'coming from or connected with the sea or lake,' an alleged reference to the dwelling place of the soul in ancient

> Northern European cultures (the numerous cultic objects and indeed human and animal sacrifices found in Northern bogs and mires may attest to this). [...] *Psyche,* [...] has links with the Greek *psykhein* 'to blow, cool' as well as various terms for life-force, ghost, spirit and even butterfly. [...] The Latin *animus,* on the other hand (often in the early centuries a translation for *psyche*), again has a variety of meanings connected with rationality, mental life, personhood, etc. It in its turn is related to the Greek *anemos*/ἄνεμος, 'wind or breeze,' and possibly the Sanskrit [word for] (ánila/'air, wind') and its cognate with the Welsh *anadl*/'breath' and Old Irish *animm*/'soul'.
>
> (Tyler, 2016, p. 13)

With this note in mind regarding the origins of the word, I will review the manner in which Plato described the body and soul, before tracing Plato's influence on the development of early Christian thinking. Although in later chapters I will particularly be focusing on Teresa of Avila and Edith Stein who were also influenced by the Abrahamic faiths, and Christian tradition in particular, in this chapter I will also touch upon Celtic spirituality, since it has also shaped my ongoing approach and interest in the relationship between the soul and the Divine. As Tyler points out,

> [O]ur description of soul reflects our deeper metaphysical views on the nature of the cosmos. Soul-language implicitly betrays our perspective on the universe (even the refusal to use the term 'soul' betrays a metaphysical perspective in itself). From Plato onwards speculation about the nature of self has automatically been connected with speculation as to the nature of the cosmos.
>
> (Tyler, 2016, p. 13)

Although Western ways of being can rightly be criticized for their historic focus on the individual and individuation, rather than a celebration of community, extended family, love of mother earth, and growth through connection, much of the more recent interest in spirituality in the West appears to be related to thinking beyond the limits of individualism and toward an interest in understanding humanity's connection to the natural environment and the rest of the cosmos. There has also been a corresponding interest in Celtic spirituality/Celtic Christianity, with its roots and incorporation of influences from Celtic pagan beliefs, which celebrate the intertwining of spirituality within nature.

A Tentative and Flexible Timeline of Contributions to the Language, and Interest in, the Soul

I have found it helpful to use a timeline on which to place the philosophers, theologians, and psychologists who have contributed various understandings of the relationship between body and soul, and the closely related concept of 'self'. Keeping in mind that it is not possible to provide firm dates for the beginnings and endings of historical periods, since competing interests in different parts of the world have shaped when the identifying aspects of a particular period might have taken hold, these following dates might be helpful to those readers new to these ideas. I have focused on the authors and bodies of work which have primarily attracted my interest in the language of the soul, while also indicating those whose work have made significant contributions and are perhaps more widely known, also acknowledging I am unable to mention everyone who has made a contribution. I will end by touching upon recent popular authors and their books, for it is clear that the interest in the soul and spirituality is not going anywhere, despite the lessening interest in organized religion.

Ancient Greek Philosophy: Socrates (470–399 BCE), Plato (428–347 BCE), and Aristotle (384–322 BCE)

Nelstrop, Magill, and Onishi (2009) suggest Plato is the best known of the ancient Greek philosophers and the most important philosopher of all time. This idea is hard to refute when realizing that his ideas continue to shape much of how we think about ourselves. Plato wrote in the form of dialogues between himself and his teacher, Socrates, and it was in his first book, *Phaedo*, that he described the human person as being made up of a physical body and a more mysterious soul/*psyche*. His descriptions, which were later referred to as "Platonic dualism" (Tyler, 2016, p. 9), are the beginning of the distrust of the body, which he suggests thwarts the nobler pursuits of the soul; the body is attracted to the worldly delights while the soul/*psyche* is drawn toward true reality. He goes on to suggest that katharsis involves a separation of body and soul, which is the aim of true philosophers, and which ultimately comes about through the death of the body. Tyler (2016) explains that for Plato the *psyche* exists before it dwells in a body and continues to exist after the body dies, being capable of several reincarnations (p. 31). Tyler points out that in his first book, Plato also describes the 'World soul' (*nous*) and *daimones,* which are like guardian angels providing a link between individuals and the gods.

It is in his second book, *The Republic*, that Plato uses the analogy of a cave as a way to describe the manner in which the body hinders the soul in its pursuit of knowledge. Plato's cave is described as connected to the outside world by a long narrow passage. Within the cave are a row of prisoners facing the wall, chained in such a way that they can only look forward to the wall of the cave. Behind the prisoners is a fire which creates light so as to cast shadows on the cave wall, and for the prisoners these shadows are their reality rather than merely shadows of objects behind them. Plato suggests that if a prisoner were to become free and turn around, all would be confusing, and particularly blinding and painful if that prisoner were to make it all the way outside into the sunshine. However, the escaped prisoner would become accustomed to natural sunlight and realize their previous limitations. Plato suggests philosophers need to realize the deceptions of the 'taken-for-granted's with which the majority of people live, strive for the soul's ascent to a greater knowledge of reality, but then be willing to return/descend again and live with the prisoners. Nelstrop, Magill, and Onishi (2009) add that this second descent after the initial ascent is also found in Christian mysticism (p. 25). Interestingly, my colleagues and I have been finding in our research on spirituality and post-traumatic resilience in relation to COVID-19, that people who are relying on spirituality to cope with the unknown of the pandemic are also describing a calling to help and serve others who may not be managing as well as they are: To these participants and to many authors, spirituality and knowledge are not only for the individual's betterment but to be used in service of others also.

In *The Republic*, Plato moves beyond the dualistic to the description of a tripartite soul, building on descriptions used in *Phaedo* of the desires within a person for food and drink, for example, and how logic needs to control these. In addition to logic and desire, a third element of will/spirit is added to the other two parts of the *psyche*/soul (Tyler, 2016, p. 34). However, his thinking and descriptions continue to evolve and become more complex in his third and fourth books, *Phaedrus* and *Timaeus*. In *Phaedrus*, he adds the role of *eros*, interpersonal love, and the development of character, alongside the reiteration of the message inscribed at the Delhi temple: "know thyself" (Tyler, 2016, p. 37). In *Timaeus*, there is a description presented of the connection between the individual soul's intelligence and the "World soul" (*nous*), so that the universe's intelligence is reflected within each individual soul (Tyler, 2016, p. 43).

I have only touched upon Plato's conceptions of the soul briefly, and have admittedly relied on secondary sources, because my aim in this chapter is merely to gesture toward the influences on ongoing discourses regarding the soul. I am hoping that even this brief outline shows that Christian theology was not the creator of the dualism of body and soul, nor the distrust of the body and its desires. Plato, through his written dialogues with Socrates, paved the way for these ideas, which certainly influenced Christian thought and Western thought more generally. However, Plato also articulated and further circulated the idea of needing to know oneself, that although the body has desires, the soul is also made up of logic and will, and that the soul is connected to something greater than itself, all of which are ideas that have continued to influence conceptualizing of the self/soul over time. Of course, Plato was not the only Greek philosopher to influence the development of Christian and Western thought; as Tyler (2016) highlights, Aristotle also has had long-lasting effects, and he argued the body is an essential element, without which the soul cannot develop and move toward perfection (p. 49). It is useful to keep these creative tensions in mind as I move on to consider the early stages of the development of

Christian thought as the Christian church moved into a less marginalized position and writers began to reflect upon the relationship between the self/soul and the Divine.

The Patristic Age (100–700 CE): Augustine (354–430 CE)

Augustine was born in Alexandria, becoming a Bishop within the early Christian church in Northern Africa in 396 CE. Although I have suggested in the last chapter that it is possible to consider two different strands within early Christianity, where one could be described as involving the desert mothers and fathers who decided to pursue a less mainstream and organized version of their faith, and the other as involving the leaders of the Church, Nelstrop, Magill and Onishi describe Augustine in such a way that he could be considered as straddling these two traditions at this time. They suggest Augustine was one of the founding fathers of Christian mysticism and explains his work, *Confessions*, "is often regarded as the first ever spiritual autobiography" (Nelstrop et al., 2009, p. 67). In this autobiography, Augustine records events in his life before his conversion to Christianity, and then moves on to represent his conversion and his understanding of the soul and the cosmos in a conversation with his mother, who was also a Christian. In a manner which foreshadows later authors of Christian mysticism and spirituality, Augustine describes the way in which he and his mother engaged initially with reflection (using the intellect) and dialogue but were required to move beyond their rational understanding to enter their souls, where they were able to encounter God: Regions of "inexhaustible abundance [... where] life is the wisdom by which all creatures come into being" (Augustine in Nelstrop et al., 2009, p. 67). Reflecting on this journey toward the encounter with God, Augustine suggests this turn toward interiority involves discovery of selfhood, resulting in his description of his understanding of the various elements of the self, or soul. While Plato offered an image of the tripartite soul, Augustine builds on this as he is also being influenced by his understanding of the Christian Trinity. He suggests that the soul has three functions, or aspects: The intellect, the memory, and the will. "Just as God the Trinity has three personas who are all interrelated within one another, so the soul, who is God's image, has three interrelated aspects" (Nelstrop et al., 2009, p. 71).

Tyler argues that Augustine has shaped an image of the soul which has cast "a long shadow on the next millennium of Western psychological development" (Tyler, 2016, p. 48). Augustine grew up in the last stages of the Roman Empire, and, having been raised by a pagan and a Christian parent, embodies "the struggles of one world ending (late paganism) and a new one emerging (medieval Christianity)" (2016, p. 67) – I wonder whether in the future our current age will also be considered as a pivotal moment as we are grappling with how we need to change and respond to the challenges of the COVID-19 pandemic and the environmental crisis.

Tyler goes on to say the struggles Augustine experienced resulted in a convoluted struggle to express his image of the soul. Although Augustine was influenced by Platonists, and by Plotinus in particular, he was also shaped by the writings of St. Paul and other Christian writers, so Augustine attempts to distinguish his Christian concept of the self/soul from the Platonic influences and context in which it developed. These various influences result in Augustine's distrust of the body and human nature, believing them corrupt and our soul's only chance for ascension coming from "God's grace". This was in contrast to "'Pelagian' notions of what we would nowadays refer to as 'original blessing'" (Tyler, 2016, p. 69).

With this difference in mind between Augustine and Pelagius, I will turn to comment upon Celtic spirituality.

Celtic Spirituality/Christianity: Pelagius (354–418 CE) and the Synod of Whitby 664 CE

Although the Celts and Celtic spirituality today might be most associated with Ireland, Wales, and Scotland, Chadwick (1970) explains "the Celtic peoples of the British Isles formed a part of the great Celtic peoples who occupied and ruled a large part of Europe before the conquest by the Romans" (p. 8). She admits the Celts of Britain and Ireland have "left the most complete picture of their civilization, having enjoyed freedom from foreign, especially Roman, conquest longer than their continental neighbors – and in parts escaped it altogether – and thus preserved their own culture in a purer form" (p. 8). Although there are difficulties in pinpointing the origins of people in space or time, especially when threads of the stories reach back into a pre-literate past, she does say, "to Greek and Latin writers of the second half of the first millennium B.C.E. [sic] the Celts were recognizable as a cultural entity occupying part of Europe" (p. 17). They gradually wandered further west and the Celtic Fringe is now recognized as referring to the "Celts of Brittany, Britain and Ireland" (p. 18).

Although academics have pointed out that the terms "Celtic Christianity" and "Celtic spirituality" are both somewhat misleading since there was no unified Celtic church separate from the Roman church of the time (Davies & O'Loughlin, 1999; O'Loughlin, 2000), it is quite fascinating that there continues to be such an interest in Celtic spirituality and a sense of it having key principles that were in opposition to the mainstream Christian/Roman church of the time and which could be recovered now. Bradley (2003) – who has remarked he would prefer now to replace the term "Celtic Christianity" with "early indigenous Christianity of the British Isles" (p. v) – suggests the Celts have a great deal to teach us about "our relationship with the rest of creation as well as with our fellow human beings. Quite alien to them was the idea of domination" of the earth (p. 58). He goes on to say,

> A recovery of the Celts' ability to find God's love and glory reflected throughout the natural world is going to be essential if we are to save our planet from environmental destruction. But scarcely less important for us today is a return to that other long neglected theme of Celtic Christianity – a view of human nature as not being radically tainted by sin and evil, intrinsically corrupt and degenerate, but as imprinted with the image of God, full of potential and opportunity, longing for completion and perfection.
>
> (Bradley, 2003, pp. 59–60)

Bradley also offers that there are many similarities between what I will continue to refer to as Celtic Christianity and the Eastern churches, with movement of people and ideas between Egypt, Syria, and the British Isles. He states that the British monk, Pelagius, traveled to Rome, North Africa, and Palestine, in the early 5th century, where he probably formulated his more "affirmative doctrines about the human condition that were to land him in such trouble with the Roman authorities [... The] British heresy of Pelagianism in fact originated in the East and found its most enthusiastic disciples among the Celts in the far west" (p. 11). Bradley points out that the biggest crime that Pelagius probably committed, alongside another Celtic theologian, John Scotus Erigena, was to challenge Augustine's doctrine of "original sin and total depravity" (p. 52). Celtic Christianity, with its influences from Celtic pagans and Druids' nature mysticism, shares much in common with North American and Australian Indigenous spirituality (p. 53).

A gathering of church leaders at the Synod of Whitby in 664 CE has been described as a key event in the further stifling of Celtic Christianity and greater domination of the organized Roman Church. At this time, King Oswin, who was more supportive of Celtic approaches in Northumbria in the North of what is now known as England, was married to a princess from the south of the British Isles who was a Roman Christian, and since the two traditions celebrated Easter at different times of the year there was a desire to streamline the church calendar. With the Roman tradition winning the debate, the Celtic ways began to retreat further, but not altogether. Nonetheless, Bradley suggests that although Whitby was the beginning of the end of distinctive Celtic Christianity in Britain it continued to flourish in many more remote areas for another 500 years and actually continues today in many smaller pockets.

To reiterate, what is most significant for my current project is the fact that although Augustine's conceptions of the human person and the soul have had a long-lasting impact, there was a competing and more positive view of the human soul presented by those supporting the Celtic tradition. This tradition also saw a close intertwining of the Divine within all of creation and not only within the human person. Although the Iona, Northumbrian, and Aidan and Hilda communities all actively promote a

Celtic form of Christianity today, Bradley worries we are in another Dark Age, where we are brutalized by the pressures within a "consumer society with its rampant acquisitiveness and selfishness" (2003, p. 119). He goes on,

> We have a long way to go, however, in recovering the Celt's wonderful and all-embracing sense of every part of the world and every aspect of life being filled with the presence of God. If we do recover it in time, perhaps we will yet save the planet that we have so nearly destroyed.
>
> (Bradley, 2003, pp. 119–120)

As O'Donohue also states in describing Celtic wisdom,

> The body has had such a low and negative profile in the world of spirituality because spirit has been understood more in terms of the air element than the earth element. The air is the region of the invisible; it is the region of breath and thought. When you confine spirit to this region alone, the physical becomes immediately diminished. This is a great mistake, for there is nothing in the universe as sensuous as God. The wildness of God is the sensuousness of God. Nature is the direct expression of the divine imagination.
>
> (O'Donohue, 1997, p. 50)

It is important to hold onto this respect for the physical – nature and the human body – as the language of the soul is re-introduced to psychology and psychotherapy and integrated into the postmodern practice of narrative therapy, which I will take up again in chapter six as I discuss Merleau-Ponty's contributions. This respect for the physical allows for the possibility of considering the spark of the divine in all things and recognizing the thinness of the veil that separates this physical world from the spiritual world (Bradley, 2003, p. 37). This has the potential for reinvigorating awe and curiosity regarding all elements of life.

Middle Ages (Triggered by the collapse of the Roman Empire between 376 and 476: 700–1500 approximately. The Early Middle Ages are sometimes referred to as the Dark Ages)

I will not say very much about the Middle Ages, wishing primarily to point out that Thomas Aquinas (1225–1274) lived in Italy during this time and was a primary figure in Christian theological and philosophical thought. Sheldrake points out that it was during the 12th century that intellectual and theological inquiry developed within schools connected to cathedrals in cities which "gave birth to the great European universities" (2013, p. 87). He describes this movement as involving more than just a shift in geography from countryside to city since universities were primarily for teaching and learning, resulting in theology focusing more on the mind and less on spirituality and its integration within an ordered or monastic life. Thomas Aquinas, as a monk within the Dominican order whose members were actively involved in education, believed that the intellectual life was a spiritual life. It was the Dominicans, including Thomas Aquinas, who "led the way in exploring how to cope theologically and spiritually with the rediscovery of Greek philosophy, especially Aristotle" (p. 87).

Thomas Aquinas was canonized in 1323, and Edith Stein, whose work I will discuss in chapter five, was to be influenced by him in some of her later work, which is why I mention him and place him within this timeline.

Reformations: Protestant and Catholic (1500–1700)

The Reformation was a period in which there was growing criticism of organized religion (the Roman Catholic church at that time) in a manner perhaps not too dissimilar to many current-day concerns. This resulted in the development of Protestant churches, led by Martin Luther in Germany, John Calvin in France, and Henry the VIII in England (although Henry's concerns could be described as more political in nature). Sheldrake indicates that it was in the 16th century that Protestant reformers were decrying "the curriculum and focus of late medieval universities – because it seemed to prepare students in a form of theology devoid of spirituality" (Sheldrake, 2013, p. 87).

What has previously been called the "Counter Reformation" occurred within the Roman Catholic tradition involving people within this tradition responding to their own and the Protestants' concerns about how the Roman Catholic church was living out its faith. One result of this Catholic reformation was Ignatius of Loyola (1491–1556) founding the Jesuits (The Society of Jesus) in France in 1540, with a commitment to spirituality and intellectual pursuits. He also developed the *Spiritual Exercises,* which I mentioned in the introduction.

At a similar time, Teresa of Avila (1515–1582) was busy in Spain reforming the Carmelite monastic tradition. I will devote the next chapter to Teresa of Avila so will not say anything about her here, other than to point out she was born and lived in Spain at a time which straddles the very end of the Middle Ages and the beginning of the Reformation period. As I will discuss in the next chapter, this was an exceptionally interesting time and place. Equally influential, was a good spiritual friend of Teresa's: John of the Cross (1542–1591). He also lived in Spain and is perhaps best known for his poem, titled 'The Dark Night', and his image of the 'dark night of the soul', which Stein was to reflect upon in detail in her final book which was to be published posthumously (Stein, 2018).

While Puritan spirituality began in England, it is perhaps best known for having emigrated to North America as early as "1620 where [Puritans] founded the colony of Massachusetts as a utopian Christian Society" (Sheldrake, 2013, p. 124). At a similar time, George Fox (1642–1691) was influenced by Puritan spirituality and founded the Religious Order of Friends, or Quakers. "He differed from Puritans in believing that humans were essentially good rather than sinfully depraved. He also taught the presence of the divine 'Inner Light' within every person and the sense of inward peace that followed from this" (p. 125). Quakers engage in silent common worship, waiting for God to lead them to speak, and a form of decision-making based upon consensus. Although grounded within an interior experience, Fox also believed this form of connecting with God would lead to eradicating human conflict and working toward transforming the social order (p. 125).

Sheldrake explains that the Reformation period was not truly complete until about 1700, by which time a third form of spirituality had arisen beside the more ordered/intellectual and mystical types, which he calls "the 'active-practical' type that emphasized finding God in everyday life and the practical service of other people – creating a spiritual climate favorable to lay Christians" (2013, p. 112). His description of this active-practical type of spirituality resonates with that of Celtic spirituality and will be called to mind in Teresa of Avila's work.

Finally, although not writing about spirituality or theology, it was during this period that French Philosopher René Descartes (1596–1650) coined the phrase "Cogito, ergo sum", or "I think, therefore, I am" in his book *Discourse on Method* (1637) (https://www.britannica.com/topic/cogito-ergo-sum). This phrase has had a lasting impact on Western discourses and debates about the position and importance of the intellect, thought, and reflection. With this, I will turn to the next period, Early Modernity, including the Age of Reason.

Early Modernity/Age of Reason (1700–1900)

Sheldrake suggests writing on spirituality is sparse during Modernity as compared to other periods, but that much of what was going on would spark what was to flower in the late 19th and early 20th centuries. However, he speaks to the broad cultural climate in Europe and North America:

> the Enlightenment, the political revolutions in France and America, and the Industrial Revolution. These are the foundations of what is often described as Modernity. The pre-Modernity world, in which religion dominated not only spiritually but politically, socially, and intellectually, gave way to a new world in which independent human reason came to dominate.
>
> (Sheldrake, 2013, p. 147)

He goes on to explain that the mid-17th century Enlightenment had its origins in the late-medieval period's Nominalism; this urged a separating of faith from reason, resulting in a split between theology, faith, and spirituality on the one side and philosophy and science on the other. He describes Europe as having been exhausted by religious conflict and fanaticism, and so detaching from tradition and authority, and moving away from "the experiential into rationalism and objectivity" (p. 147).

German philosopher Immanuel Kant (1724–1804) is considered an Enlightenment philosopher and I will touch on his influence in phenomenology within the chapter about Edith Stein. Sheldrake describes Kant as seeking a religion without revelation – although some might call him an agnostic or religious skeptic. Sheldrake says of Kant,

> He was certainly not an orthodox Lutheran but, by cutting the ground from under traditional metaphysics (i.e., by denying that we can have *knowledge* of realities that transcend nature) and invalidating the classic proofs for God's existence, he claimed to be making proper room for faith rather than the opposite. What drove his religious vision was neither natural theology nor mysticism but conscience which, Kant asserted, alone teaches the reality of a righteous God who will vindicate the claims of moral justice. In this perspective, religion effectively becomes ethics.
>
> (Sheldrake, 2013, p. 148)

During this period, a distinctive American form of spirituality also developed, which was shaped to a certain degree by the mentality associated with the concept of the American Frontier. Sheldrake is clearly not referring to the Indigenous spiritualities in North America as he focuses on describing the settlers' mentality: "The frontier mentality, with its rough and ready lifestyle – not to mention a stark symbolism of living on the margins where the forces of good and evil confront each other – provided fertile ground for numerous evangelistic revivals" (p. 167). Nonetheless, back on the East coast of North America, in New England, experience interwove with aspects of the Enlightenment "and literary-poetic sensibilities to give birth to American Transcendentalism" (p. 167), of which Ralph Waldo Emerson (1803–1882) is considered a primary figure. Emerson distanced himself from classical Christianity, drawing upon Hindu scriptures also. This "led him to a position of non-dualism and to espouse the unity of the human soul with the surrounding world [which sounds similar to Celtic and Indigenous spiritualities and the idea of 'World soul' (*nous*)]. Other influential themes included his emphasis on individuality, human freedom, and self-reliance [which sound much more similar to a typical American rugged individualism associated with the frontier mentality]" (p. 168).

Modernity to Postmodernity (1900–2000) (Postmodernity Beginning Post WWII)

The transition from Modernity to Postmodernity is considered to have occurred in relation to a growing realization that relying on human reason had not solved problems nor answered questions, and, in fact, some would suggest, had been the foundation from which atrocities like the Holocaust had arisen. During this time, the birth of psychology also drew attention to the complexity of human nature. Two world wars occurred, and the atomic age demonstrated "human technology was capable of catastrophic destruction" (Sheldrake, 2013, p. 174). This was not the first period to experience political unrest and wars, but global travel and communication brought about rapid change. The Civil Rights Movement began in the United States of America, and social change and women's rights were raised in the Northern Hemisphere. Building upon these descriptions, Sheldrake says,

> "Postmodernity" therefore defines a culture where the simple answers and optimism of a previous age are impossible. By the close of the twentieth century, previously fixed systems of thought and behavior had fragmented, and the world was understood as radically plural. People had become increasingly suspicious of normative interpretations of truth. In Western societies as well as globally, cultural, religious, and ethnic diversity was increasingly identified as the fundamental reality of human existence.
>
> (Sheldrake, 2013, p. 175)

Correspondingly, during this time, attendance at organized religious settings declined, and a growth in inter-religious dialogue began. Christianity, alongside other religions, became more global, although much of the newer enthusiasm for Christianity was centered within the global south where it has particularly been tied to Gustavo Gutiérrez (1928–) and Liberation Theology.

An interesting and influential French Jesuit during this period was Pierre Teilhard de Chardin (1881–1955). He was both a scientist – paleontologist – and mystic, who attempted to bridge the gap between science and spiritual teachings. I mention him as his work inspired the version of the 19th annotated approach to the *Spiritual Exercises* (Savary, 2010) that I completed which I mention in the introduction, as well as due to his vision of spirituality.

> Teilhard embraced a fundamental optimism whereby evolution became a mystical and cosmological principle. Humanity is not alienated from but embedded in the material order, and, with the world, progresses both forward in an evolutionary sense and "upward" towards God. [...] Teilhard also sought a kind of mysticism of involvement in the world, both inanimate and animate, [...].
>
> (Sheldrake, 2013, p. 191)

Here, again, is the idea that spirituality should not be considered only an insular and individual form of mysticism, removed from the world, but as intimately connected to the cosmos and involved with the rest of the world.

Thomas Merton (1915–1968) is another key figure during this period whom I have mentioned in the last chapter. He was born in France, educated in England, but is probably most associated with Gethsemani Abbey in Kentucky, USA, where he lived as a Trappist (reformed Cistercian) monk and followed the Rule of St. Benedict. Sheldrake describes Merton as contributing to the reintegration of spirituality into theology during this time; he is remembered for his "contribution to Christian-Buddhist dialogue, and for his later commitment to issues of social justice and world peace" (Sheldrake, 2013, p. 184). So, again, spirituality is not only about quiet individual withdrawal from the world but should result in a recommitment to a shared responsibility for the future of humanity and the world.

As Sheldrake also points out, it is difficult to know at this point which of the philosophers, theologians, psychologists, and writers who are hard to place within a discipline, will be remembered as the most significant in the future when people look back. Nonetheless, I wish to name those who have contributed to discourses of the soul/self in this period, so as to be clear as to their placement on this timeline.

Nelstrop, Magill, and Onishi (2009) describe American philosopher and psychologist William James (1842–1910) as the father of the modern study of mysticism, or spirituality. He published a series of lectures in 1902, titled *The Varieties of Religious Experience: A Study in Human Nature*, in which he described mystical states of consciousness. James was most interested in individual and personal experience of religion versus organized religion; and, reacting against Kant's claim that we cannot know God because our senses and reason cannot experience the Divine, "James postulates the existence of a faculty in human beings that is deeper than the senses – which allows an intuitive grasp of reality beyond that which the evidence of our senses can provide" (Nelstrop et al., 2009, p. 4). He suggests that these mystical experiences have four characteristics, the first two being of greatest significance: ineffability, noesis, transiency, and passivity. Ineffability refers to the manner in which an altered state of consciousness, which might be experienced in a spiritual experience or as a result of anesthesia, cannot be put into words and described to anyone who has not had a similar experience. His descriptions relied on writers like Pseudo-Denys and are similar to the '*via-negativa*', as mentioned in the last chapter, where paradox assists in moving beyond the limitations of naming and conceptualizing (Nelstrop et al., 2009, p. 5). Noesis is described as a flash of inspiration and related to a sense of oneness with all things (Nelstrop et al., 2009, p. 5). Transiency recognizes that mystical/spiritual experiences are usually fleeting, and passivity refers to the sense of one's personal will being surrendered to, or overwhelmed by, a higher power. (These descriptions are similar to Engler's descriptions of self and 'no-self', also described in the last chapter.)

Sigmund Freud (1856–1939) has had a profound and lasting effect on Western society, resulting in many ways of thinking about the human person that have taken on the status of 'truth's, or 'taken-for-granted's. However, concepts such as the ego, id, and superego as parts of a person's self are merely *one* way of conceptualizing a structure of the self and are ideas that came about within a particular time and place about 100 years ago. It would be impossible to do his ideas justice in a few short paragraphs here, so I will limit myself to Tyler's report on the context in which Freud's work was translated and the impact of this on the language of the soul. Tyler points out that psychoanalysis was presented to an American audience at the Mental Hygiene Congress in 1930 within the context of a new movement needing to prove itself respectable. Otto Rank presented at the congress and spoke to the differences between a scientific and a human approach to understanding human behavior, arguing that psychoanalysis was scientific, despite the fact more recent critiques of Freud's work would suggest it was not informed by a scientific methodology (Tyler, 2016, pp. 99–100). It was within this same context that James Strachey, who translated Freud's work from the original German to English, preferred to "invent Greek or Latin equivalents that sounded a little more medical or specialized" (Tyler, 2016, p. 107) in order to argue for psychoanalysis's worth to American and British scientific and medical communities. Although in the original German, Freud referred to "*Ich, Es* and *Über-ich* (literally 'I', 'It' and 'Over-it' [...], Strachey uses the terms 'ego', 'id' and 'superego'" (Tyler, 2016, p. 107). Freud was reportedly not happy with this translation, preferring simple pronouns to remain connected to popular ways of thinking and to make these ideas more available to patients. Tyler goes on to point out that simple terms such as "slip of the tongue (*Fehlleistung*)" and "the unknown thing" become "the parapraxis" and the "unconscious" respectively. Yet, the shift in language is argued as being most apparent in relation to Freud's language about the whole self:

> Freud's preferred terms are *die Seele, seelische* and *Seelenleben,* literally, 'the soul', 'soulish' and 'soul-life', all of which Strachey replaces with 'the mind', 'mental' and 'mental life'. The effect of this, argues Bettleheim, is to replace Freud's 'direct and always deeply personal appeals to our common humanity' with 'abstract, highly theoretical, erudite and mechanized – in short, "scientific" – statements about the strange and very complex workings of our mind'.
>
> (Tyler, 2016, p. 108)

For Tyler, the battle over the 'soul' within psychoanalysis is also seen more broadly in the struggles within psychoanalysis and psychotherapy in the debates about how much the clerical/religious and/or medical professions were to dominate. Calling upon Bettleheim again, he points out that the medicalization of Freud's language overly focuses on the rational mind and loses Freud's focus on the emotional and spiritual/soulish elements of a person.

Before continuing to follow the trace of psychoanalytic thinking on the language of the soul, I want to briefly mention that Edith Stein (1891–1942) can be considered a contemporary of Freud's. Her work on understanding the person was developing alongside his and was therefore not directly influenced by his theorizing, which I find refreshing. She did begin her university education with a focus on psychology as she studied with William Stern (1871–1938), but quickly switched her focus of interest to Edmund Husserl's (1858–1938) phenomenology. She has been described as someone whose interests at one point might have been met in modern day's study of psychiatry, but after her conversion her work became more that of a Christian philosopher. I will describe her work in detail in chapter five.

Maurice Merleau-Ponty (1908–1961) was a French phenomenological philosopher who was also influenced by Husserl. He incorporated his interest in the body into phenomenology as he wrote about the role of embodied perception in meaning-making, linking art, psychology, language, and religion, which I will explore in chapter six. Mikhail Bakhtin (1895–1975) was a Russian philosopher of language, literary theory, and ethics, whose work and influence David Crawley will be describing in chapter seven.

Returning to psychoanalysis and the language of the soul on this continuing timeline, Carl Jung (1875–1961) has been described as someone who was "entirely comfortable in his own version of neo-Gnostic spirituality" (Tyler, 2016, p. 10), developing Jungian psychology in such a way after his split from Freud as to incorporate an element of the transcendent. However, it was James Hillman (1926–2011) who took back the language of the soul more fully. Hillman's early career was as the leader of the C.G. Jung Institute's study program before leaving Zurich to pursue academic study and the development of a theory of 'archetypal psychology'. Becoming disillusioned by academia, his next step was to set out to develop "ecopsychology", drawing upon the neo-Platonic ideas of the "World soul" (*nous*) (Tyler, 2016, p. 122) – which can be considered consistent with Celtic-spirituality's focus on the divine within nature. He then began to write more for a popular, rather than academic, audience as he wrote his successful *The Soul's Code: In Search of Character and Calling* and appeared on Oprah Winfrey's television program. Although Tyler focuses primarily on Hillman's more academic texts, I am always also interested in popular cultural texts which appear to capture the popular imagination since these often seem to speak to broad concerns and interests within the general public, which often also show up in the therapeutic context.

Tyler highlights that Hillman's aim was to restore the soul (*psyche*) to psychology, and that Hillman argued that both psychology and academia had removed the soul from its proper place. Hillman's aim then was:

> To restore the mythical perspective to depth psychology by recognizing the soul's affinity with, nay love for, the Gods … Or, as the

> Greeks may have said, to reaffirm the tragic connection between the mortal and the immortal, that natural plight of the soul that lies at the base of any psychology claiming to speak of psyche.
>
> (Hillman in Tyler, 2016, p. 123)

Indeed, in *The Soul's Code: In Search of Character and Calling*, Hillman's reliance on Greek philosophy and Plato is further evidenced. He begins by making several statements which are initially engaging, and I can imagine why they have had broad appeal. For instance, he starts chapter one by saying, "There is more in a human life than our theories of it allow" (Hillman, 2017, p. 3). Consistent with a narrative therapy stance, he suggests, "Our lives may be determined less by our childhood than by the way we have learned to imagine our childhoods. We are [...] less damaged by the traumas of childhood than by the traumatic way we remember childhood" (p. 4). He suggests that repair will come about by focusing on the power of character and personal calling – that sense of purpose or reason for being alive. Also consistent with a narrative therapy approach, he implies it is both boring and unengaging to only focus on the problem storyline (although he does not use that term), "itemizing events [...]: This came after That. Such a life is a narrative without plot" (p. 5). He goes on to say that we have dulled our lives by the manner in which we have thought about them, and he argues for bringing romance and fictional flare back into our lives, by considering ideas such as beauty, mystery, and myth.

Admittedly, despite being able to imagine how these beginning pages might inspire a general and broad audience, it is possible to already note something that Tacey critiques in Hillman's work. Hillman is already suggesting that everyone has a destiny written inside themselves just like there is "destiny written into the acorn" (Hillman, 2017, p. 5). The acorn's destiny is to be an Oak tree, and we, according to Hillman, need to allow ourselves to be led by our *daimones* (Plato's term), spiritual guides, or soul companions, to allow for the unfolding of our characters and allow ourselves to be drawn into our true calling. I will discuss how Stein discusses unfolding in chapter five. However, there is something of the American focus on individual success and happiness that appears to be called upon in some of Hillman's descriptions, as if he is suggesting that if only we give ourselves over to our true selves, we will live successful, happy, fulfilling lives. Tacey, from a Jungian perspective, also says,

> While Hillman criticizes Jung for being a dualist, it is James Hillman who, in the last analysis, is the ultimate dualist, because he can never reconcile inner and outer, psyche and society, ego and underworld, therapy and activism … Hillman's inability to grasp paradox leads to the disastrous outbreak of overt contradiction.
>
> (Tacey in Tyler, 2016, p. 126)

Tyler prefers to use a Wittgensteinian perspective and "criticize Hillman for holding a somewhat illusory and probably indefensible notion of 'inner' and 'outer', 'us' and 'them' [...] that cannot be reconciled within the system that he is proposing" (Tyler, 2016, p. 126). (Ludwig Wittgenstein [1980–1951] was born in Austria and studied philosophy in England. Tyler describes the impact of Wittgenstein's work and the postmodern turn, particularly in relation to his ideas about the "way of seeing" [Tyler, 2016, p. 155.]) In going on to provide an example of Hillman's traditional understanding of soul as "an inner place or deeper person or ongoing presence" (Tyler, 2016, p. 126) and Hillman's description of interiorizing as moving from the outside visible surfaces to a deep invisible place, Tyler shows Hillman's constraint by dualistic thinking, which is something which postmodern narrative approaches attempt to avoid. Nonetheless, Hillman's project to bring the soul back into psychology certainly speaks to a popular interest in the soul that is continuing to fascinate people.

M. Scott Peck's (1936–2005) book, *The Road Less Travelled: A New Psychology of Love, Traditional Values and Spiritual Growth,* was first published in 1978, with the 25th-anniversary edition published in 2003. It has reportedly sold more than 7 million copies, although I have only recently been inclined to read it to see what all the interest was about. Peck was an American psychiatrist who described himself as not belonging to any particular school of psychotherapy; "I am not simply a Freudian or Jungian or Adlerian or behaviorist or gestaltist" (p. 12). However, he does call upon Freudian concepts considerably and also says, "Freud, a rationalist and scientist par excellence, [...] and since he is the most influential figure in modern psychiatry (for many good reasons), his attitudes have contributed to the concept of religion as neurosis" (p. 207). This comment has traces of Tyler's arguments as presented above – Freud's work was definitely taken up in America, and by this American psychiatrist, as scientific and distanced from religion, faith, and spirituality. Despite this, Peck provides examples of the importance of faith and spirituality in his patients' lives. Relying a great deal on Jungian dream work and long-term psychotherapy, he comments in his preface that he believes brief approaches, although helpful, are superficial. This is an unfortunate comment at a time when few people can afford to pay for private long-term psychotherapy, and socially funded agencies are required to limit the number of subsidized appointments available to each service user. More often than not, agencies today are also offering brief and single sessions in walk-in contexts. As a colleague, Joanna Bedggood, has pointed out, some psychotherapists might condescendingly refer to these services as 'band-aid solutions', but sometimes band-aids are very useful. People are actually able to accomplish a great deal more than some might expect in a short period, perhaps focusing on specific goals, developing a focus on resilience, and strategies for connecting to naturally occurring supports.

Nonetheless, Peck's book is divided into four sections: Discipline, Love, Growth and Religion, and Grace. He argues for a return to good 'sensible' parenting to instill self-discipline and ego boundaries in children. He also suggests there is no distinction between mind and spirit "therefore no distinction between the process of achieving spiritual growth and achieving mental growth. They are one and the same thing" (p. 11). This idea appears to contain traces of Aquinas' belief that the intellectual life is a spiritual life, as described above. However, I found Peck's final book section focusing on grace the most liberating of the four sections, offering an approach that is more consistent with narrative interests in alternative and preferred storylines in addition to problem storylines.

It is perhaps not unexpected that this book would have been so successful with an American audience where there was already more of an interest in psychotherapy and self-help than there originally would have been in England at the time, for example – although this interest in psychotherapy may have been expanding globally more over the past 25 years. The section on grace has Peck examining those times when despite childhood histories and expectations of problems, good things happen, people succeed and flourish. He talks about the "miracle of serendipity" (p. 243) and then goes on to describe the "miracle of evolution" (p. 263). Some of what he says resonates with Teilhard de Chardin's concept of evolution and his "law of the attraction-connection-complexity-consciousness [...] that is giving evolution its direction" (Savary, 2010, p. 17). However, what I find more challenging are Peck's comments that are summed up as he says we are "growing toward godhood" (p. 270), and "The idea that God is actively nurturing us so that we might grow up to be like Him brings us face to face with our own laziness" (p. 271). This idea of becoming godlike resonates to a certain degree with descriptions of mystical union with the Divine in the inner mansions of the soul in the work of Teresa of Avila, John of the Cross, and Edith Stein. However, in Peck's writing I wonder how these ideas contribute to the popular interest in his book, and if they are building upon a North American Protestant work ethic and a focus on personal development.

Thomas Moore (1940–) is also American, a former monk and university professor, and a practicing psychotherapist, influenced by Jung and Hillman. His book, *Care of the Soul: A Guide for Cultivating Depth and Sacredness in Everyday Life,* was first published in 1992 and has reportedly sold over 1.5 million copies. The 25th edition was published in 2016. Moore is described as often being on television and radio programs, "most recently on Oprah Winfrey's *Super Soul Sunday*" (back book cover). His book is divided into four sections: Care of the Soul, Care of the Soul in Everyday Life, Spiritual Practice and Psychological Depth, and Care of the World's Soul. (I mentioned Moore in this chapter's introduction as I described his project of returning 'soul/*psyche*' to psychology, psychiatry, and psychotherapy.) He calls upon Plato's descriptions of Socrates's comment, "I do nothing other than urge young and old to care not just for their persons and property, but more so for the well-being of their souls" (Plato in Moore, 2016, p. XIII). He builds upon this as he describes himself as offering private consultations which he refers to as 'psychotherapy',

> but [...] in the Platonic sense – service to or care of the soul. The main difference between psychotherapy in the usual sense and mine is the emphasis on matters of the soul rather than managing a person's life and resolving problems and emotional tensions. It isn't that I don't want to help a person navigate the knots we all get into in relationships, dealing with past trauma, and finding purpose. It's more that I want to honor what is presented and let it offer the potential good it holds. I don't want to be a problem-solver of emotions.
>
> (Moore, 2016, p. XXIV)

This description sounds oddly similar to a narrative approach, in which 'problem-solving' is not the main focus either. As narrative therapists, if we engage with people in such a way as to highlight their values, hopes, and preferences, and if we demonstrate curiosity regarding what is 'absent but implicit' in their complaints (as described in chapter one), problems have a tendency to dissolve; White particularly describes how this can come about by scaffolding conversations and supporting movement from what is 'known and familiar' to what is 'possible to know' (White, 2007).[1] I have written previously (Béres, 2014) about how liberating this can feel, since we do not need to have all the answers nor feel required to become experts in problem-solving. As people are supported in trusting their own expertise, prior knowledge, and skills, and in articulating their values, hopes, and dreams, they begin to develop their own solutions. What Moore offers is another way of looking at this as perhaps being related to caring for the person's soul.

Moore argues that spiritual health is as important as physical and emotional health, simultaneously describing his own redefinition of religion for himself. He is not interested in religion as creed, dogma, or moral persuasion, but rather in religion as depth of meaning, which results in "a sensitive ethical response to the world. Respect for the mysterious is, to me, the heart of religion" (Moore, 2016, p. XXVII). This underlying framework has him describing care of the soul as being about giving ordinary life depth and value – which resonates with Celtic spirituality and White's interest in the 'spirituality of the surface' and 'little sacraments of daily existence' (described in chapter one and mentioned above). Moore says, "'Soul' is not a thing, but a quality or a dimension of experiencing life and ourselves" (2016, p. 5). In a similar vein to Hillman's interests, and building upon Plato's notion of 'World soul' (*nous*), Moore also describes caring for the soul of the world as well as our own and others' souls. He critiques modernity's focus on an inanimate world and inanimate objects, where "*Inanimate* means 'without *anima*' – no *anima mundi*" (Moore, 2016, p. 268). He goes on to say that modernity's paradigm suggests people "*project* life and personality onto things" (p. 268), which he argues provides the ego far too much power. He says,

> My own position changes when I grant the world its soul. Then, as the things of the world present themselves vividly, I watch and listen. I respect them because I am not their creator and controller. They have as much personality and independence as I do. [...] Everyone knows that we can be deeply affected by the things of nature. A certain hill or mountain can offer a deep emotional focus to a person's life or to a family or community.
>
> (Moore, 2016, pp. 268–269)

I appreciate Moore's descriptions of a person's soul and of 'World soul' (*nous*), and also appreciate his focus on the *care* of these souls. Acknowledging and describing soul is not merely a theoretical exercise for Moore, but also results in a nurturing two-way relationship.

Conclusion

While I was in the process of researching and writing this chapter, *Soul* (Rivera, 2020) won an Oscar for best animated full-length movie, which seemed serendipitous as I have been arguing for the fact that people continue to be fascinated by the idea of soul. Even within this animated movie, some of the various ideas and discourses I have been tracing across the past 2,500 years in this chapter surface as ongoing popular ways of imagining soul. The story in *Soul* presents iridescent young souls being prepared to enter physical bodies on earth, and other older (still iridescent) souls leaving bodies and progressing upwards on what looks like a heavenly conveyor belt to what is suggested is Heaven. However, the story focuses on a particular soul, Joe, attempting to return to his body on earth after its death because he does not want to miss out on what he imagines would have been his big break into the type of life that was going to bring him a sense of meaning and purpose, after a successful audition as a jazz and blues pianist (even the music has soul). In fact, there is much time spent on the idea that the little baby souls who are being prepared for their bodies on earth need to first find their spark – what will give them meaning and purpose in life. However, by the end of the movie, the message is presented that people have spent too much time worrying about what is to give them a sense of meaning and purpose and rather we should focus more on enjoying the world – nature, sunshine, pizza, and lollipops, and being curious about one another: A reminder, again, to keep our feet on the ground as we pursue the language of the soul.

In this chapter I have presented an argument that the language of the soul is rich with complexity and we do well not to remain stuck at the point of Platonic dualism, merely separating the spiritual or iridescent soul from the worldly physical body. The language of the soul includes descriptions of the body, the intellect, memory, and will, as well as connections with the 'World soul' (*nous*), and the ability to engage in wonder, appreciation, and awe – which then calls for a response of care and action. I believe this language assists with the postmodern narrative focus within therapeutic contexts of opening up space for conversations that move toward what is 'possible to know' from what is 'known and familiar' and toward 'preferred storylines' from 'problem storylines'.

Note

1 This idea of "problem dissolving" is related to Wittgenstein's approach to the "dissolution of philosophical problems" (Kuusela, 2019). Wittgenstein's later work, which has had long-lasting effects, straddling modernity and postmodernity, was regarding ways of seeing. Tyler (2016) explains that Wittgenstein's work in this area was based upon his prolonged reflection on Jastrow's 'Duck-Rabbit' diagram. In relation to the simple diagram that some might initially see as representing a duck and others might see representing a rabbit, Wittgenstein was fascinated by how nothing about the diagram changes while at the same time everything about how it is perceived might change. Disillusioned by logic and scientific attempts at describing cause and effect, he also is disinclined to understand the shift in perception by a turn to inwardness and an examination of something that some might call the unconscious.

References

Béres, L. (2014). *The narrative practitioner*. Palgrave MacMillan.

Bradley, I. (2003). *The Celtic way. New Edition*. Darton, Longman & Todd.

Chadwick, N. (1970). *The Celts*. Penguin Books.

Davies, O. & O'Loughlin, T. (1999). *Celtic spirituality*. Paulist Press.

Hillman, J. (2017). *The soul's code: In search of character and calling*. Ballantine Books. (Original work published 1996.)

Kuusela, O. (2019). On Wittgenstein's and Carnap's conceptions of the dissolution of philosophical problems, and against therapeutic mix: How to solve the paradox of Tractatus. *Philosophical Investigations*, *42*(3), 213–240. DOI: 10.1111/phin.12227.

Moore, T. (2016). *Care of the soul: A guide for cultivating depth and sacredness in everyday life, Twenty-fifth anniversary edition*. Harper Perennial. (Original work published 1992.)

Nelstrop, L. with Magill, K., & Onishi, B. B. (2009). *Christian mysticism: An introduction to contemporary theoretical approaches*. Ashgate.

O'Donohue, J. (1997). *Anam cara; A book of Celtic wisdom*. Cliff Street Books, an imprint of Harper Collins Publishers.

O'Loughlin, T. (2000). *Celtic Theology: Humanity, World and God in Early Irish Writings*. Continuum.

Peck, M. S. (2003). *The road less travelled: A new psychology of love, traditional values, and spiritual growth, Twenty-fifth anniversary edition*. Touchstone. (Original work published 1978.)

Rivera, J. (Producer), Docter, P., & Powers, K. (Co-Directors). (2020). *Soul* [Animated Movie.] United States: Disney & Pixar.

Savary, L. M. (2010). *The new spiritual exercise: In the spirit of Pierre Teilhard de Chardin.* Paulist Press.

Sheldrake, P. (2013). *Spirituality: A brief history, Second Edition.* Wiley-Blackwell.

Stein, E. (2018). *The Science of the Cross.* (J. Koeppel, O.C.D., Trans.) ICS Publications. (Original work published in 1983.)

Tyler, P. (2016). *The pursuit of the soul: Psychoanalysis, soul-making and the Christian tradition.* Bloomsbury T & T Clark.

White, M. (2000). *Reflections on narrative practices: Essays and interviews.* Dulwich Centre Publications.

White, M. (2007). *Maps of narrative practice.* W.W. Norton.

4 Teresa of Avila's Interior Castle

Laura Béres

Having presented a 'broad strokes' overview in the last chapter of how the soul has been considered and described over the past 2,500 years in primarily Western discourses, I will move on in these next three chapters to focus on specific writers whom I have found helpful in assisting with my project of introducing the language of the soul to narrative therapy. In this chapter, I will explore Teresa of Avila's (1515–1582) descriptions of the soul. Although she discusses the soul in her *Autobiography* (*Life*), *Meditations on the Song of Songs* (*Meditations*), and *The Interior Castle* (*IC*), Williams (1991) points out that ten years separated her writing of *Life* and her writing of *IC* in 1577. During this time, she had been busy with the Carmelite Reform and also experienced the impact of the Spanish Inquisition. He says themes that were already there in her earlier work are more deeply rooted and more clearly expressed in *IC*, which is why I will focus primarily on *IC* although I will draw upon *Meditations* also. Williams particularly points out that Teresa is clearer in *IC* about what needs to be avoided on the soul's journey, i.e., "the religiosity of a private self" (p. 113), going on to say *IC* is "among other things an attack on interiority as an ideal in itself" (p. 116).

Teresa of Avila's style of writing is informal and chatty as if she merely wrote down what she was saying aloud to her fellow nuns. Her sentences run on and she often uses self-deprecating remarks as she describes herself as a simple uneducated woman with no ability to write clearly who will require men of superior intellect to correct any errors she might have included. These remarks can seem excessive and somewhat distracting, especially for someone in the 21st century with feminist sensibilities, yet they appear to go hand in hand with Teresa's insistence regarding the importance of humility and the transformative process possible if a person is willing to gain self-knowledge and to commit to contemplative prayer. She writes like a caring spiritual director providing advice as to how to engage in this process, along with suggestions as to how to discern whether experiences are truly of God and how these experiences should result in loving acts. She argues that any interior spiritual journey must be balanced with a commitment to showing God's love in community, bringing together the Biblical images of both Mary, who sat mindfully at Jesus' feet,

DOI: 10.4324/9781003137450-7

and Martha, who busied herself in the kitchen working to provide hospitality to the guests in their home.

To ground my discussion of Teresa's concept of the soul, I will refer again to Lydia, whom I described in chapter one. After Lydia had indicated that she was feeling much more content and peaceful about her decision to stop attending church because she was tired of being 'preached at by middle aged white men', she decided to discontinue counseling for a while, as services transitioned from in-person to online due to restrictions and guidelines as we all responded to the spread of COVID-19. However, five months later, Lydia contacted me again and asked to recommence counseling due to what she described as increased anxiety. Since we were experiencing a third wave of high numbers of cases of COVID-19, we recommenced our sessions online. She indicated she thought her anxiety was primarily in response to this third wave and the corresponding third 'stay at home' order. In asking her if she had been able to maintain some of the activities that she had previously developed and described as having 'fed her soul', she admitted she had not. She said she was battling herself to a certain degree as she told herself what she knew she should do – such as walk more or integrate some exercise – but she could not motivate herself. She indicated that everything was going well at home with her husband, son, and daughter, but, as a self-proclaimed extrovert, she said she was missing her friends. Having discussed this, and asked her about what difference it might make to think in terms of loving herself and thinking of what her soul needed, rather than using her willpower to try and do what she thought she 'should' do, she returned to a follow-up appointment saying that this shift in thinking had made a great deal of difference. She said it was easier to get out of bed and do some yoga if she thought of this as a form of showing love to herself, whereas if she told herself she 'should' do that, she was more likely to rebel against this suggestion and stay in bed longer. However, in that same follow-up session she also indicated that she continued to worry about her anxiety, so I shifted into an externalizing conversation with her about the anxiety. She was able to describe both anxiety and insecurity as two characters in her life who seemed to shift places with each other, with one taking more of a role in her life as the other stepped back. Merely speaking in terms of Lydia not being the problem, but rather "the problem being the problem" resulted in Lydia saying, "that is very helpful". In examining the effects of anxiety she clearly indicated not valuing any of the effects – this was not the sort of anxiety that might make her work harder, for instance, but rather would have her withdrawing from experiences due to fear – she was able to realize that she actually valued freedom, and so did not like how anxiety was limiting her choices. I raise Lydia's situation again here prior to moving on to Teresa's description of the soul as layered, because I think Lydia highlights how multilayered people are, and how, even when interested in their soul and spirituality, they obviously continue to be fully present in the world with all its preoccupations. Their attention and focus will shift back and forth between these various aspects of themselves and their worlds.

I will turn to a description of my approach to engaging with Teresa's ideas about the soul, some of the recent interest in her writing, and explain the time and context in which she was writing. I will then present her metaphor of the soul as a castle with many mansions, her descriptions of the faculties of the soul and the related image of friendship.

My Approach

I have already described my overall approach to the study of the language of the soul in chapter two, but I have specifically engaged with Teresa's work on the soul in three different ways: I have read English translations of her own writing which was originally published in Spanish; I have read academics' commentaries on her work; and I have attempted to experience what she wrote about in my own contemplative prayer practice and within spiritual direction. As Tyler (2011) points out, Wittgenstein's method of "aspect seeing" provides a useful approach to understanding the strategies of the mystical writers such as Teresa (p. ix). Applying Wittgenstein's approach to the spiritual realm he suggests,

1 Everything that can be put into words can be put clearly
2 Philosophy will signify what cannot be said by presenting clearly what can be said
3 There are, indeed, things which cannot be put into words. They make themselves manifest. They are mystical. (Drury in Tyler, 2011, p. 47)

Later he describes Wittgenstein's and Teresa's approach as a "threefold path of saying-showing-acting" (Tyler, 2011, p. 182). In a similar vein, in his chapter about mystical affinities between Teresa and Jean Gerson, Tyler points out that Teresa said of the process of contemplative prayer outlined in *IC* that she could not explain the process in the inner mansions, but would rather have to show it, which she did in her style of writing. He quotes Teresa as saying there are things in the inner mansions of the soul "which the understanding does not have the capacity to grasp […] although […] those who have experience, especially a lot of it, will understand very well" (Teresa in Tyler, 2017, p. 42). Tyler points out how Dionysius's explorations regarding the importance of eros on the spiritual path would have influenced Osuna and Gerson, both of whom influenced Teresa. Eros is described as a different form of knowing than that which comes about by mental effort, or as Gerson would put it, "it is a knowing which involves the libidinal or *affectus* as much as the *intellectus*" (Tyler, 2017, p. 45). Hence my approach to Teresa's work on the soul through an attempt to experience through practice and *affectus* as well as through the intellect. This approach has resulted in focusing on what Teresa says and implies about the structure of the soul (as layered, and with faculties), the complexity of what she describes as the center of the soul, and her use of the image of friendship.

Recent Interest in Teresa's Work

Writing in 2015, at the time of the 500th anniversary of Teresa of Avila's birth, Odell has responded to the question of what a 16th-century female mystic might offer contemporary women of faith. Having sought input from female academics, Gillian Ahlgren, Mary Frohlich, Elizabeth Dryer, Julia Feder, and Katie Bugyis, Odell argues Teresa is described as a marvel who "taught the meaning of humility in the Christian life" (2015, p. 2a), whose view of women as having "spiritual merit, gifts and talents pushed against the norms of her day" (2015, p. 2a). She goes on to quote Bugyis as stating, "today's women understand how hard it was for Teresa. Five centuries later, women still fight to be accepted on the basis of their gifts and talents" (2015, p. 2a). Teresa, therefore, speaks to women who, despite the differences in the 21st century, continue to experience a lack of equality in terms of being accepted for who they are in religious and secular contexts.

Mujica describes the far-reaching influence of Teresa's work in the contemporary world. For instance, she describes "popular self-help writer Caroline Myss [as having] created a small industry around Teresa with her *Entering the Castle* books and CDs" (Mujica, 2010, p. 16), as well as new books appearing in France, Germany, Italy, and Spanish speaking countries. She indicates that contemporary popular writers have suggested that Teresa is "a mystic for our times" (Mujica, 2010, p. 16), although she argues that to fully appreciate the significance of Teresa's work it is important to understand her as a woman of her own times. She focuses on Francisco de Osuna's *Third Spiritual Alphabet* and its influence on Teresa in regards to the importance of interiority and stillness (Mujica, 2010, p. 16), conjuring up the image of the hedgehog curling up in on itself, since this is an image Teresa uses and is where the image originally came from. She then goes on to describe the ever more heightened tension today between organized religion and personal faith or spirituality, which she suggests results in many people turning "to New Age Cults to satisfy their spiritual longing, unaware that their traditional religions do offer an alternative to the mechanized rituals" (Mujica, 2010, p. 17). As touched upon in chapter two, this dissatisfaction with Christian religion in the West has also resulted in Westerners looking to the East for alternative practices. She describes Mirabai Starr, translator of a 2008 edition of the *IC,* who is of Jewish background but a practicing Buddhist, as seeing a similarity between Buddhism's notion of the fundamental emptiness of all phenomena and Teresa's teaching (Mujica, 2010, p. 18). This suggests that contemporary people searching for an alternative to the "mechanized rituals" in religion might be just as attracted to Teresa's *IC* as they are to mindfulness practices within Buddhism. Despite this, Teresa's "teachings are firmly rooted in Catholic doctrine and, indeed, she called herself a 'daughter of the church'" (Mujica, 2010, p. 18). Tyler (2013) also describes these similarities and differences between Buddhism and Teresa's form of prayer.

Tyler relates Teresa's form of prayer to the "contemporary discourse on mindfulness, especially as adapted from the Buddhist tradition" (Tyler, 2013, p. 184). He points out how contemporary healthcare and psychotherapy have been drawing upon Buddhist sources as they have integrated mindfulness into their health and social care practices. He highlights the purpose of Buddhist informed mindfulness as being the development of a detachment from the "entanglement with things as they seem" (Tyler, 2013, p. 187). Although he explains the differences in Teresa's method of prayer, he also explains that where her account converges with Buddhist mindfulness is in "the importance of drawing attention away from the intellectual and mental activity to the location of what she calls 'the heart'" (Tyler, 2013, p. 190). In fact, Teresa's descriptions of beginning to practice her form of contemplative prayer suggest that in the initial stages it can be difficult to quieten the distracting thoughts and fears, just as it is difficult to quieten them in the beginning stages of practicing mindfulness, yet says, "In enabling these souls to overcome their initial difficulties, the Lord has granted them no small favour, but a very great one" (Avila, 2013, p. 38). This also shows the importance of humility again as she does not believe overcoming these difficulties is due to anyone's skills, but rather due to grace and a willingness to let go of reliance upon the intellect.

In reviewing these recent descriptions of how people are engaging with Teresa of Avila's teaching I am underscoring the fact her work from the 16th century does, indeed, inspire fascination from a variety of academics as well as people looking for meaningful spiritual practices in the 21st century. Feminists may be interested in her as a role model for engaging in spiritual practices when women's ways continue to not be fully respected. At the same time, people seeking spiritual practices that are less controlled by Church structure may be drawn to her descriptions of interior contemplative prayer leading to a potentially unmediated union with the Divine. Nonetheless, it is possible to gain a more thorough understanding and appreciation of her teaching if we also understand the context of her work.

Teresa's Life and Times

Teresa was born in Spain in 1515 and died there 67 years later in 1582 (Ahlgren, 2016, p. xiii). She became a Carmelite nun, entering the monastery of *Encarnación* in Avila in 1535, which was "far from the ascetic desert envisaged by the first Carmelite fathers and later reformers" (Tyler, 2013, p. 62). Tyler describes Teresa as being central to a group who gathered there to discuss the need for them to live a simpler religious life – suggesting the founding of a group of "shoeless – *Descalza* sisters" (2013, p. 66), and leading to Teresa's "'great project' of reform based on the lives of the 'holy fathers of old'" (2013, p. 66). She was a Prioress during this time of reformation, was canonized in 1622, and was the first woman named Doctor of the Church in 1970 (Avila, 2013, backcover). In *St John of the Cross*, Tyler provides a helpful description of the "perceived 'oddness' of Spain" (2010, p. 9) which had such a profound impact on both Teresa of Avila and then John of the Cross (1542–1591), whom he describes as having developed an "easy spiritual rapport" when they met in 1567 (p. 18).

Tyler (2010) explains Spain's unique history as being distinct from the rest of Europe. Shortly after the beginning of Islam in 711, Arabs defeated the Christian kings of Spain and occupied much of northern Spain by 714 (Tyler, 2010, p. 9). The new government promised freedom of worship to Jews and Christians and established an atmosphere of reconciliation, with intermarrying between the groups (Tyler, 2010, p. 10). However, "[b]y 1085 the so-called Christian Reconquista or 'Re-conquest' of Muslim Spain reached a significant turning point when the ancient capital of Toledo was retaken" (Tyler, 2010, p. 10). The Christians gradually consolidated their lands over the next four hundred years and by the time Ferdinand and Isabella became "Their Catholic Majesties" in 1492 the end of "eight hundred years of Muslim, Christian and Jewish interaction on the Peninsula" (Tyler, 2010, p. 10) was essentially marked. Shortly before this, in 1478, the Spanish Inquisition was formed for the expulsion "or forced conversion of Spanish Jews" (Tyler, 2010, pp. 10–11). From then onwards, Spain attempted to homogenize, celebrating pure Christian lineage while developing a growing suspicion of "'New Christians' or conversos" (Tyler, 2010, p. 11).

During these times of suspicion and control in Spain, for a relatively short period, from the late 15th century into the beginning of the 16th century, the Franciscan Cardinal Cisneros encouraged the publication into Spanish of many mystical texts from the late Middle Ages making these "available for lay-people, including women" (Tyler, 2010, p. 13). Teresa's uncle made sure Teresa, as a young woman, was able to benefit from these texts (Tyler, 2017, p. 36) which had a profound influence on her, but by the time she was a mature woman and wanted to provide these books to the nuns in her convents, they had been "prohibited by the Valdés Index" (Tyler, 2010, p. 13).

Tyler (2013) describes the impact the Holy Inquisition and Jewish Spain would have had upon Teresa and her work. Although for many years Teresa had been considered as having come from a long line of Christians, evidence was found in 1946 which showed that when Teresa's father and his brothers attempted to prove their noble blood (Tyler, 2013, p. 30), in order to avoid a new tax, testimonies actually showed that Teresa's grandfather had been a convert from Judaism. Testimony was provided indicating that while he lived in Toledo he had been required to wear "a garment of humiliation that those tried by the Inquisition had to wear as they processed through the streets for public ridicule" (Tyler, 2013, p. 31). It was following this humiliation that the family moved from Toledo to Avila, where they lived in great wealth, having made their money in the cloth and silk trade (Tyler, 2013) and presented themselves as having a pure Christian lineage. Tyler argues that this context needs to be considered when reading Teresa's work

Teresa of Avila's Descriptions of the Soul

As a Castle with Many Mansions/Rooms

Teresa says she was instructed by a superior in the Carmelite Order to write a book about her form of prayer, and having beseeched God to speak through her, she began to think "of the soul as if it were a castle made of a single diamond or of very clear crystal, in which there are many rooms, just as in Heaven there are many mansions" (Avila, 2013, p. 3). She goes on to say that since God created us in His image and likeness, and since we cannot fully comprehend God, it is also not possible for us to be able to attain a full comprehension of our "soul's great dignity and beauty" despite how acute our intellect may be (p. 4). In this way, she appears to be choosing to focus on the beauty of the soul as being made in God's image and likeness rather than privileging discourses regarding the sinfulness of the soul – which is more consistent with doctrine associated with Pelagius rather than Augustine, both of whom were discussed in the last chapter. Yet, Teresa immediately goes on,

> As to what good qualities there may be in our souls, or Who dwells within them, or how precious they are – those are things we seldom consider and so we trouble little about carefully preserving the soul's beauty. All our interest is centered in the rough setting of the diamond, and in the outer wall of the castle – that is to say, in these bodies of ours.
>
> (Avila, 2013, p. 4)

She is suggesting the body is the outer aspect of the soul, and that the soul is not something static and unchanging, waiting to be discovered lurking in our depths. She suggests, rather, that the soul is complex and that we can either ignore it or choose to pay attention to it, developing practices, such as contemplative prayer or mindfulness, that may support its further refinement.

Teresa says the soul, as a diamond or crystal castle, "contains many mansions, some above, others below, others at each side; and in the centre and midst of them all is the chiefest mansion where the most secret things pass between God and the soul" (Avila, 2013, p. 5). Williams (1991) explains this idea of the self turning in and entering itself in prayer was fairly common, and that Teresa was aware of this at the same time as she was aware of the lack of clarity with this idea. She attempts to provide some clarification of the process precisely by using the image of the castle, explaining how this turning inwards to find the Divine at the center, involves choices as we muddle about in this labyrinth of mansions. Williams points out Teresa is anxious to alert us to our liability to make mistakes:

> [T]he 'interior castle' is an image of the richness and variety of the soul considered as the dwelling place of God; but it also points at the teasing and even perilous character of the inner world, where we cannot instinctively find our way. There is, of course, an initial 'cleaning of the glass' to be done by turning away from the mortal sin that can darken the soul, though it can never extinguish the fountain of light at the centre.
>
> (Williams, 1991, p. 114)

Teresa explains we need to turn away from a preoccupation with worldly affairs and worries about how we are perceived and toward self-knowledge; we need to become aware of the vastness and complexity of our soul as an interior castle yet not focus on self-knowledge for self-knowledge's sake, but in order to orient ourselves and turn toward an "awareness of its true relation to God: it must acquire self-knowledge understood as humility and repentance" (Avila, 2013, pp. 114–115). Williams explains that directing the mind to the self and to its perfection keeps a person tied to the self, whereas the purpose of Teresa's type of contemplative prayer is to become free of the self and rather bound to God.

Teresa appears to be suggesting in the second chapter of her first mansion that self-knowledge and humility go hand in hand and that since the intellect cannot possibly comprehend all there is to know of the soul and the soul's relationship to God, "it is through the abundant mercy of God that the soul studies to know itself" (Avila, 2013, p. 14). Recognizing the limit of our intellect and our need to rely on a higher power can help foster humility.

In the only chapter of the second mansion, Teresa again stresses the need to engage in conversations with good people, reading of good books, and listening to good sermons as a way to cultivate our ability to listen to God, who will speak to us more directly when we are in the innermost mansion of our soul. This could suggest a social constructionist, or Foucauldian-like, recognition of technologies of the self, where there is a realization of the impact on self of the activities we choose to engage in and the discourses within which we immerse ourselves: a recognition of the social construction of identity, as described in relation to narrative therapy in chapter one.

Teresa presents a picture of the soul as being something different from the physical body, but certainly embodied. She describes the soul as vast and lofty and although she says we "must not imagine these mansions as arranged in a row, one behind the another" (Avila, 2013, p. 13), she also describes them as if they are layered: the soul turns its attention from the outside, entering the first mansions through prayer and self-knowledge and then with God's assistance moving further through the mansions to the center where the soul abides with God. Prayer will be experienced differently within the different mansions as the soul continues to be more easily distracted by the outside world in the first mansions and distracted by different forms of worries and fears and frustrations in other mansions. Although the will and intellect will assist with prayer and focus in the earlier mansions, they are more apt to hinder the development of humility and so also hinder progress toward the center mansion. This perhaps is similar to Lydia's realization that attempting to use her will and intellect and telling herself she 'should' do something was not having the effect she wanted.

Edith Stein, whose work I will discuss in the next chapter, also describes how it is possible in meditation or prayer to attempt to focus the mind and then become aware of the mind wandering, but how, in addition to this, it seems as if there is another part of the self watching the wandering mind (Stein, 2000). (In a similar way, Tyler describes the Buddhist idea of "monkey mind" [Tyler, 2013, p. 86].) In attempting Teresa's form of contemplative prayer, this process can also be discerned. Tyler says much more about the similarities and differences between Buddhist 'no-self' and Teresa's descriptions of the soul in this form of Quiet Prayer that she is describing in *IC*, which I will come back to.

The Soul's Faculties

In some of the earlier mansions described in *IC*, the mind seems very busy and can become distracted by its own thoughts (Lydia described the thoughts triggered by anxiety as leading to "catastrophizing" also), but Teresa tells us in the first chapter of the third mansions that we need to keep persevering in "detachment and abandonment of everything" (Avila, 2013, p. 40). In the following chapter of the third mansions she points out that not only do we need to stop relying on our intellect, but we also need to give up our will, and rather want God's will to be done. In this way, we are provided with a picture of the soul not only as a castle with many mansions but also as having certain faculties such as intellect and will which we will need to let go of in the journey to the center and toward God. She also says, "let us leave our reason and our fears in His hands and let us forget the weakness of our nature which is apt to cause us worry. Let our superiors [in a Convent setting] see to the care of our bodies; that must be their concern: our own task is only to journey with good speed so that we may see the Lord" (p. 46).

Williams' commentary on Teresa's writing is helpful as he explains, despite having denied any distinction between "soul" and "spirit" in *Life*, she admits in the fourth mansions of *IC* that she needs to differentiate them in some way. She says that she was encouraged by a learned man, whom Williams suggests might have been John of the Cross, to "separate 'mind' or 'imagination' (*pensamiento* or *imaginación*) from 'understanding' (*entendimiento*): the imagination can run loose even when the intellect or understanding is in touch with God" (Williams, 1991, p. 123). He explains this is important as it highlights a difference between the conscious mind within the earlier mansions and what can happen in the "depths of the self" (p. 123). He goes on,

> the conventional threefold division of the soul is breaking down in the Castle: instead of the three faculties on the same plane enjoying different degrees of 'union' with God, the intellect's absorption standing alongside the imagination's mess, Teresa is looking for a model that allows her to talk about different levels of a more integrated mental-spiritual action: 'the soul is perhaps completely joined with them in the dwelling places very close to the centre while the mind is on the outskirts of the castle suffering from a thousand wild and poisonous beasts' (IV, 1.9).
>
> (Williams, 1991, pp. 123–124)

Each time I read Teresa's writing something new captures my interest (my imagination?). As I recently have been re-reading it for clues as to her ideas about the soul, beyond the metaphor of a diamond castle, her comments about the soul's faculties have become more obvious to me. These ideas may have been 'taken-for-granted' for her, and as Williams points out, she was not particularly interested in developing a coherent structure for the soul, but rather explaining and showing her form of quiet contemplative prayer. Nelstrop, Magill, and Onishi (2009) describe how later medieval accounts of the soul, having been influenced by Augustine, also developed:

> The notion that the soul is made up of different aspects is a fundamental element of later accounts of mysticism. We noted Augustine did not see intellect, will and memory as separate faculties but interrelated aspects that are only truly the image of God through their participation in God. Yet as the Middle Ages progressed something of the subtlety of Augustine's argument appears to be lost as intellect, memory and will are increasingly treated as a mimetic, rather than a participatory, image of the Trinity. […] attention shifts to consideration of the spark of the soul within the conscience. Later writers increasingly come to view intellect and will as separate faculties, with defined relationships to lower faculties, such as sensation and imagination.
>
> (Nelstrop, Magill, & Onishi, 2009, pp. 72–73)

Certainly, when we turn to Edith Stein's work we will see this development further, but this is also descriptive of Teresa's accounts. In the fourth mansions, Teresa says, for instance, "I came to understand by experience that thought (or to put it more clearly, imagination) is not the same as understanding" (Avila, 2013, p. 57). She goes on by wondering why understanding, as one of the "faculties of the soul" seems so timid compared to thoughts and she adds, "It exasperated me to see the faculties of the soul, as I thought, occupied with God and recollected in Him, and the thought, on the other hand, confused and excited" (p. 58).

As Tyler says, "one of Augustine's chief contributions to the Western understanding of self is his division of the soul into memory, understanding and will" (2016, p. 73). These terms are perhaps not used in the same way today, however, and he points out that memory for Augustine is "more than just a faculty of recollection: it really means the whole mind, both conscious and unconscious, in contrast to mind – [...] which refers only to the conscious mind" (Louth in Tyler, 2016, p. 73).

The Complexity of 'Center'

Returning to Teresa's use of the metaphor of a diamond castle made up of many mansions for the soul, with different faculties, we see she also describes the center/seventh mansions of our soul, as we turn inwards and silence our thoughts, letting go of a need to understand, allowing God/the Divine to draw us further into communion with Him. Just as faculties and diamond castles may not be metaphors that fit together smoothly, so the idea of the center of the soul does not hold up to the intellect's exploration of it. I have begun to imagine the center of the soul as something more like a black hole, or wormhole, as we are drawn to the center where we could theoretically imagine an opening up to the vastness of the universe, or of the Divine.

Returning to Tyler's account of the similarities and differences between Buddhist "no-self" and "mindfulness", and Teresa's form of prayer in relation to the "center" of the soul, he says, "Teresa has thwarted expectations in a way only she could do. The intellectual, analytic or discriminating mind wants a 'centre' or 'essence' of the self or soul. Teresa just will not deliver" (Tyler, 2013, p. 200). He explains that she says the inner depth is either an experience too sublime to be able to describe, or a call to engage in good acts, but also that the center is "Christ Himself as revealed through the meeting in the Triune God. For at the centre of the soul is 'where God Himself is'" (Tyler, 2013, p. 200). Asking, in relation to Buddhist "no-self," whether there is alternatively a "fixed self" in Teresa's writing, he replies, "There is and there isn't" (p. 201). He clarifies that for Teresa the call to the center is felt more than thought and that the fruits of such a spiritual journey to the "center" – to God – will be good works in the world. He argues that Teresa's form of prayer is as radical in its "deconstruction of the self" as Buddhist mindfulness and no-self, although Teresa is clearly Christian and focused on a personal and creative God. This radical deconstruction of the "self" while also fully embodied could, indeed, be congruent with narrative therapy's sensibilities.

These thoughts about Teresa of Avila also suggest Meister Eckhart, a 14th-century mystic, to whose work I am also drawn. He is described as enigmatic and controversial, "Christian pastor and Buddhist sage. He is a Neoplatonist and Aristotelian, prophet of feminism and ecological saint" (Davies, 1991, p. 1). He is also credited for inspiring such contemporary philosophers as Heidegger and Derrida. His use of language, which "disrupt[s] our thought patterns in order to lead us on to a higher, more essential form of knowledge" (Davies, 1991, p. 5), is reminiscent of the complexity of Derrida's work and challenges us in a similar way to Teresa as they both appear to be attempting to engage us with concepts that are similar to those of Buddhist "no-self" and "non-attachment". Tyler (2017), offering a brief description of intellective and affective Dionysianism, or negative theology, suggests Teresa is neither of these, but rather more "Gersonian" in her approach. Howells (2017), in further exploring negative theology, summarizes the six areas of Teresa's teaching that Tyler argues are similar to Gerson's mystical theology:

1 Led by the will
2 Unknown, i.e., without the working of the intellect
3 Felt affectively, often using the language of taste (*sabor, gustar*)
4 With an ecstasy told in erotic language derived from the Song of Songs
5 In the high point or spark of the soul (Teresa's preferred terms are 'centre', 'deep' and 'interior' […])
6 Best understood using a distinctively non-speculative, practical presentation (unlike the Dionysianism of Eckhart or Nicholas of Cusa) which requires plain language, an emphasis on experience, and an outflow from contemplation into active good works (Howells, 2017, pp. 52–53)

Teresa's work, although less 'intellectual' in its style than Eckhart's, appears to me to share some similarities in terms of arguing for the need to detach from thoughts and concepts. This need for detachment on the journey to this complex notion of the center of the soul is similar to notions of non-attachment and its relation to mindfulness and no-self. These ideas of non-attachment can initially appear uncaring to students and practitioners in the West. Balancing non-attachment with an understanding of interconnectivity and community rather than using a Western notion of the separate individual self, adds care back into the equation for Westerners. Teresa's descriptions of the Mary-like inner journey of Quiet Prayer is also balanced with the call to Martha-like good acts in the world. Additionally, while the center of the soul is a place of union with the Divine, which brings about a Cosmic image for me, the language of friendship also brings balance by providing a down to earth homely image of Christ as friend.

The Image of Friendship in the Soul

Williams (1991) argues that Teresa makes the ideal of friendship pivotal in her theological vision, which he says was remarkable at a time when society was much more concerned with honor.

> Friendship, so people had assumed since Aristotle, was a relation between equals, and was therefore sharply restricted in scope by a system of social honour. Teresa begins from a conviction that God has freely made us friends of God, and, on that basis, she moves easily to the model of a community in which 'all must be friends' [...] irrespective of social standing.
>
> (Williams, 1991, p. 22)

Although the Song of Songs is written 'with an ecstasy told in erotic language', I am more interested in how Teresa's meditations on the Song of Songs can be approached through her focus on friendship with God. Rodriguez and Kavanaugh, in their introduction to their translation of Teresa's *Meditations*, suggest the content of it fits into four sections:

1 Mystical experience of some words from Song of Songs
2 Purpose in writing Meditations
3 The kiss as a symbol of peace and friendship
4 Communion in friendship (Rodriguez & Kavanaugh in Avila, 1980, p. 213)

Throughout *Meditations* she then distinguishes between true and false peace and the process of moving from friendship with things of the world toward friendship with God. As she also does in *IC*, she emphasizes how Quiet Prayer and union with God will result in committing to active service as well as contemplation.

Teresa says, "in many ways does our King offer souls peace and friendship" (Avila, 1980, p. 229), but also suggests the most intimate friendship will be like that modeled by the bride in Song of Songs when she asks, "Let Him kiss me with the kiss of His mouth". She encourages people not to become discouraged, saying, "whatever the friendship you have with God, you will be very rich if there is no fault on your part" (p. 229), but immediately goes on to say we should also feel very sorry if it is our fault that causes us "not to reach this excellent friendship and that we are happy with so little" (p. 230). Reminiscent of her description of the soul's progress in prayer through the mansions of the interior castle toward union with God, Teresa describes various types, or levels, of friendship that the soul can experience on its movement toward the most intimate form of friendship, as it is more easily distracted by the world and fears in the earlier levels of friendship (such as Lydia's anxiety and catastrophizing). Also reminiscent of her description in *IC* of how the intellect cannot assist with movement into the center mansions, she describes how the faculties of the soul are not involved when experiencing the type of union with God that is exemplified in the image of bride and bridegroom, saying, "the Lord ordains that the soul function so wonderfully, without its understanding how" (p. 252).

Teresa is describing the soul's journey toward an ever-deepening friendship with God through her *Meditations* yet despite the image of bride and bridegroom, rather than diamond castle, she is presenting a description of the soul and its relationship with God which is consistent with her descriptions in *IC*. Regardless of the similarities, however, the focus on friendship with God adds an extra emphasis to the love and intimacy that is possible to experience with God in the soul, and so is all the more focused on affect rather than intellect.

Conclusion

In this chapter I have described how Teresa of Avila uses a down to earth conversational manner to write about her life and contemplative prayer experiences, giving a rich picture of her understanding of the soul and its relationship with the Divine. For her, the soul is vast and beautiful because it is made in God's image and provides a means for deepening a friendship with God, but it also needs to be nurtured. Despite her commitment to writing simply, she is writing about ideas and practices that are just as complex as Eckhart's, so they are difficult to pin down and summarize. For the purposes of this current project, however, the key points for a post-modern therapist would be: the soul is not static but can be nurtured, it can be thought of as layered, with faculties, as a way of connecting with the Divine, and is also drawn to socially just practices in the world rather than only interior mystical experiences. The fact these ideas share similarities with Eastern religions, I think makes this all the more appealing for therapists committed to working in culturally respectful manners. It is certainly possible to see why Edith Stein would have been so drawn to Teresa's writing and ideas and I will pursue how she developed these in the next chapter.

References

Ahlgren, G. T. (2016). *Enkindling love: The legacy of Teresa of Avila and John of the Cross*. Fortress Press.

Davies, O. (1991). *Meister Eckhart: Mystical theologian*. SPCK.

Howells, E. (2017). Teresa of Avila: Negative theologian? In P. Tyler, & E. Howells (Eds). *Teresa of Avila: Mystical theology and spirituality in the Carmelite tradition* (pp. 51–63). Routledge.

Mujica, B. (2010). Teresa of Ávila: A woman of her time, a saint in ours. *Commonweal*, *137*(4), 15–18.

Nelstrop, L. with Magill, K., & Onishi, B. B. (2009). *Christian mysticism: An introduction to contemporary theoretical approaches.* Ashgate.

Odell, C. M. (2015). Still a beloved friend. *National Catholic Reporter, 51*(19), 1a–2a.

Stein. E. (2000). *Philosophy of psychology and the humanities.* In M. Sawicki (Ed.). (M. C. Baseheart and M. Sawicki, Trans.) ICS Publications. (Original work published in 1922.)

Teresa of Avila. (1980). *Meditations on the Song of Songs, In The Collected Works of St. Teresa of Avila, Volume Two.* (O. Rodriguez, O. C. D. & K. Kavanaugh, O. C. D., Trans & Eds). ICS Publications. (Original work published in 1611.)

Teresa of Avila. (2013). *Interior Castle.* (E. Allison Peers, Trans. & Ed.). Random House. (Original work published in 1577.)

Tyler, P. (2010). *St. John of the Cross.* Continuum.

Tyler, P. (2011). *The return to the mystical: Ludwig Wittgenstein, Teresa of Avila and the Christian mystical tradition.* Continuum.

Tyler, P. (2013). *Teresa of Avila: Doctor of the soul.* Bloomsbury.

Tyler, P. (2016). *The pursuit of the soul: Psychoanalysis, soul-making and the Christian tradition.* Bloomsbury T & T Clark.

Tyler, P. (2017). Mystical affinities: St. Teresa and Jean Gerson. In P. Tyler & E. Howells (Eds). *Teresa of Avila: Mystical theology and spirituality in the Carmelite tradition* (pp. 36–50). Routledge.

Williams, R. (1991). *Teresa of Avila.* Morehouse.

5 Edith Stein's Conceptions of the Person[1]

Laura Béres

I have suggested, in the last chapter, that Teresa of Avila's writing presents in a down-to-earth simple manner, despite the complexity of her descriptions of the soul; reading her work is like sitting down and chatting with a friend. Although Edith Stein reports that she was influenced by Teresa of Avila, and this is clear in her later work as she references the image of the soul as an interior castle, her writing is far more complex; reading her work is like sitting in a doctoral seminar, as she leads her students into an ever more nuanced exploration of being and experience. In fact, the editors of Stein's *Finite and Eternal Being: An Attempt at an Ascent to the Meaning of Being* (*FEB*) warn that readers will need to "studiously grope" and "engage in lengthy and difficult analysis" of her text, although they will eventually appreciate the truth and beauty of her arguments once they have all come together (Gelber & Leuven, 1949, p. xxiv).

Stein has been described as controversial and paradoxical (Calcagno, 2007) and as one of the most complicated of all the saints (Tyler, 2016). She was born October 12, 1891 into a Jewish family in Breslau, which was part of Germany at that time. She claims she lost her Jewish faith in her youth and later converted to Christianity, becoming a Catholic in 1922 and then a Carmelite nun in 1933. She was killed in Auschwitz on August 9, 1942, beatified in 1987, and canonized in 1998 (Borden, 2003; Calcagno, 2007; Payne, 2000; Tyler, 2016).

Stein was writing phenomenological essays at the same time Freud was developing his psychoanalytic method. Borden (2003), therefore, suggests Stein was not influenced by him, although there may have been instances of parallel development. I find Stein's descriptions of lifepower and layers of human being interesting because she developed these ideas without the influence of Freud, when currently it is almost impossible not to be influenced by his concepts. In her later work, she carries her conceptions of human being and her study of phenomenology forward as she incorporates her deep personal faith into her work and begins to turn her attention to medieval Christian philosophers and mystics. Although Stein died prior to the postmodern period, her work not only developed in response to discourses within modernity, then incorporated medieval sources, but also

DOI: 10.4324/9781003137450-8

gestured toward discourses prevalent within postmodernity (Tyler, 2016). In this way, her work could be described as straddling pre-modernity, modernity, and postmodernity, as she offers a view of being that may add to, but also be compatible with, the theory and practice of postmodern narrative therapists.

For the purposes of this chapter, I have explored the English translations of Stein's work (originally written in German) in which she presents her conceptions of human being and the soul, focusing on *Philosophy of Psychology and the Humanities* (*PPH*) (2000), *Finite and Eternal Being: An Attempt at an Ascent to the Meaning of Being* (*FEB*) (2002), and, to a lesser degree, *Potency and Act* (*PA*) (2009). More recently I have also explored her reflections on John of the Cross in *The Science of the Cross (SC)* (2018). Nonetheless, due to the ongoing importance of the phenomenological approach and her ongoing conceptions of layers of human being in her later work, it is useful to first describe these before turning to the importance of the image of the Trinity to her understanding of human being in *FEB*. I will then present a case example before discussing her use of the image of stages of night in the process of unfolding in *SC*.

The Phenomenological Approach

Borden (2003) describes phenomenology, as developed by Husserl, as being a "rigorous method focused on how we gain knowledge" (p. 20). She suggests phenomenology can be traced back to Kant (1724–1804) and Hegel (1770–1831), but that Husserl (1859–1938) is considered the founder of the more contemporary phenomenological approach (p. 21). Both she and Sawicki (2000) argue that Husserl's phenomenological approach developed in the early 1900s as a response to two opposing approaches to knowledge and learning: David Hume's (1711–1776) Empiricism, and Idealism, or neo-Kantianism. Empiricists argue that knowledge can only be based upon an exploration of what can be seen, touched, and measured. Idealists argue that "spatiality, temporality, sequence, and the other conditions permitting us to touch and measure at all are actually even more basic than the data we receive through our senses" (Sawicki, 2000, p. XI). These overarching categories were described as "transcendental" and more appropriate targets for investigation. Borden, however, also clarifies that "Kant made a clear distinction between the phenomenal and noumenal realms, or 'mere appearances' and the things as they are in themselves", going on to say, "Phenomenology makes no such distinction, and 'phenomena' in phenomenology are not opposed to noumena" (p. 22). She provides a simple analogy, suggesting empiricists would be more likely to use a microscope to understand an objective world 'out there', whereas idealists would be more interested in focusing on understanding the microscope and how the structure of the microscope affects what we see through it. Kant claimed that when we find cause and effect relationships in the world it is because our minds (the microscope) are organized in such a way to look for cause and effect relationships. Husserl, and Stein, insisted that it was crucial to straddle these two approaches by examining the subjects experiencing the world, and also the objects in the world that they experienced (both the microscope and the bug under the microscope, as Borden puts it). This shifts the focus from merely examining consciousness and the structures of the mind, recognizing that consciousness is always of something, but at the same time recognizes that an object cannot be examined for what it is without acknowledging that it is examined and experienced by someone, suggesting the relationship between subject and object is important. "The phenomenological method is most properly a description of phenomena, and the goal is an accurate description of our experience" (Borden, 2003, p. 23). The accurate description of our experience will need to involve describing both the subject examining the object and the object, acknowledging that others might experience it differently. Using this phenomenological method, Stein came to describe her understanding of how individual humans experience objects/events, giving, as part of that, a description of the various elements of human being engaged in experiencing. I will use Gricoski's (2020) example of Edith Stein considering a cherry tree later in this chapter as a further example of this phenomenological method.

Layers of Human Being in Philosophy of Psychology and the Humanities

After transferring her studies from William Stern's psychology to Edmund Husserl's phenomenology, Stein completed her doctoral thesis, *On the Problem of Empathy*, in 1916, which subsequently influenced her ideas in *PPH*, published in 1922. These two earlier publications are not considered part of her work as a Christian Philosopher but offer hints of her openness to the possibility of God. Borden (2003) suggests a surprising number of students of Husserl's phenomenological movement came to the Christian faith, as he did himself late in life (p. 6). She argues this is because the phenomenological method requires bracketing presuppositions (recognizing and putting aside 'taken-for-granteds', as I might describe them when writing about narrative theory and practice), and an openness to considering all experience – including religious experiences – prior to making any judgment.

Sawicki (2000) clarifies in her Introduction to *PPH* that Stein does not use "person" as a synonym for "human individual". For Stein, "[h]uman being is a porous and multiply stratified way of being, and 'person' designates just one of its layers" (p. XV), which is important to remember when reading Stein's descriptions of human being. Also important is the significance of the distinction between causality and motivation in Stein's thinking. Stein recognizes that in the physical and scientific world it is often possible to describe causal relations, however, she also describes times when rational, but not necessary, connections exist between events: She suggests these are due to motivation rather than causality. Stein draws upon this distinction between the laws of causality and the laws of motivation, suggesting they each rule different elements of the human being.

Borden (2003) points out that different translators have translated Stein's terms for the four layers of human being from the original German somewhat differently, but I will use those within the Baseheart and Sawicki edition of *PPH* where they are translated as the physical, the sentient, the mental, and the personal. They are considered as different realms of a human being, each responding differently to any given phenomenon, where, as has been stated above, a phenomenon is understood as the interplay between the existence of an object or event, and the internal experiencing of it. Sawicki presents Stein's descriptions of phenomenal realms as related to physical layers of the body in the following manner:

1 The physical phenomenal realm is related to matter and the physical components/layer of the body
2 The sentient/sensory phenomenal realm is related to the responsive sentience of the body
3 The mental/intellectual phenomenal realm is related to the body's *mind*, *spirit* or intelligence, and,
4 The personal, individual phenomenal realm is related to the unique personality of a human being (Sawicki, 2000, p. XVI)

In this way, Stein is moving beyond the dualism of body and soul, placing these realms all within the body, "where all four express what is ordinarily termed the soul as well" (Sawicki, 2000, p. XV) and where each realm influences the other. In fact, the body could be thought of as part of the soul, rather than a container of the soul. I have italicized 'mind' and 'spirit' to highlight that these terms are often used in a similar manner and that spirit relates to the mental layer in this schema. Stein suggests mechanical causality rules the physical realm, sentient causality the sensory realm, rational motivation the mental realm, and personal motivation the personal realm. Each of these realms is permeable within the individual, but permeable in different ways outside of the individual. The physical realm is causally connected to the physical world but not the sentient realm of other beings, whereas the sensory realm is open to causal influence among other sensate individuals – where we might feel empathy for someone, or cringe as someone hurts themselves. The mental realm is open to motivational influences among intelligent individuals and the personal realm is motivationally connected to the world of values (an important element in narrative therapy), but not other personal beings (Sawicki, 2000, p. XVII). In other words, the human being is not a closed system. By describing this interplay of causation and motivation,

Stein stresses something that Sawicki suggests is overlooked in much of psychology as it is taught and practiced today;

> Stein would reject any psychology that proposes causal explanations for human actions solely in terms of environmental influences (as behaviourism does) or personal history (as psychoanalysis does) or genetic programming (as developmental and essentialist gender-based theories do) or chemical balances (as the pharmacological management of mood does).
>
> (Sawicki, 2000, pp. XVII–XVIII)

Each of these theories is too narrowly focused for Stein and ignores an element of human life that fascinated Stein: those times when people manage what would seem unpredictable and accomplish more than they could even have imagined themselves capable. Stein's descriptions of lifepower begin to explore this interest. In the three layers of the human, other than the personal layer, lifepower can be depleted or nourished by outside sources: "art, music, and nature can feed and replenish lifepower supplies analogous to physical rest" (Borden, 2003, p. 35). Stein also suggests that the personal layer has its own source of lifepower. She says, "the person is the power source from which the acts are supplied, and she [...] consumes her lifepower on her own (for her soul)" (Stein, 2002, p. 309).

Earlier on in *PPH*, Stein has asked, "What is this mysterious something, the soul?" (2002, p. 228). In exploring this question, she comes to a point at which she then needs to distinguish soul from mind. She initially says, "With the mind we simply take on the world, but our soul takes up the world into itself. The world 'strikes a chord' within your soul, and in a special way in each individual soul" (p. 230), but then goes on to say this separation does not hold up. She then describes the "living of the soul as mental" and the soul's being as "nonmental" (p. 230). She suggests, "Your soul's being is like the core in which it roots, an individual as such, something indissoluble and unnameable" (p. 231). I will explore these ideas further in discussing her conceptions of the soul in *FEB*, but Stein is already alluding to the complexity of these ideas, where soul can be thought of as encompassing everything about a human being and also related to the idea of a core element.

Body, Soul, and Spirit in Finite and Eternal Being

Stein had begun to turn her attention to the study of Thomas Aquinas as early as the 1920s, and so also to the project of linking his method to Husserl's phenomenological method. In her Foreword to *PA*, which was written prior to *FEB* but not published until later, Stein says that she was accustomed to the phenomenological "way of thinking, which eschews doctrinal lore" (Stein, 2009, p. 1) and so initially unsettled by the use of

Scriptural passages in Aquinas's arguments. Stein points out that the Greek and medieval philosophers were focused on questions related to the meaning of being, leading the Greeks to examine "the natural givenness of the created world" while Christian thinkers placed these questions within "revealed truths of the supernatural world" (Stein, 2002, p. 4). In drawing upon Aquinas's approach, she was attempting to remedy what she saw as a problem in modern philosophers' work, where they had lost interest in questions of being, and rather were interested in the problem of knowledge, thereby severing any link with faith and theology. This appears to be a similar project as that of Husserl's phenomenological response to Empiricism and Idealism, as it attempts to straddle two ways of looking at experience.

From having begun her career studying the experiences of finite human beings, Stein moved on to examine both finite and eternal being in *FEB*, using her unique combination of the phenomenological approach and Aquinas's scholastic method. Gelber and Leuven (1949) point out that as Stein's descriptions of finite being unfold "an original and boundless ground is revealed which leads to Eternal Being" (p. xxiii). In her Introduction, Stein states, "There is only one Truth, but it unfolds itself to our human perspectives in a manifold of individual truths" (Stein, 2002, p. 1). Stein suggests Aquinas assists with this project of recognizing the manifold of individual truths, and how the in-depth study of any one individual truth may open up "enlarged vista[s]" (p. 1). Any experience can be studied from either the finite or infinite perspective; if studied from the finite (human being), as Stein engages with it, the work could be considered that of a Christian philosopher, if from the infinite (Divine), that of a theologian (Gilson, 1952; McInerny & O'Callaghan, 2016).

Having translated Aquinas's *Disputed Questions*, and studied his work carefully, Stein completed *Potency and Act (PA)* as her *Habilitationsschrift*, a book, or second doctoral dissertation, for the application process to become Professor. Her application was not to be successful due to Nazi politics at the time, and the publication of *PA* was to be delayed until many years after her death, but her understanding of potency and act was to provide a foundation in Part II of *FEB* for the exploration of finite being compared to infinite being. Potency, possibility, or the potential to act in certain ways, is compared to a being's actions. Whereas she suggests God's potency is active rather than passive, and so He is always acting (even if an action is His choice not to intervene), human being's potency and act may evolve, which she comes back to later in her descriptions of the soul.

Moving on to Part VII of *FEB*, The Image of the Trinity in the Created World, Stein suggests the image of infinite Being/God as Trinity will provide a useful image for understanding experiences of finite being. She uses Aquinas's term, saying God as Triune is hypostasis, or underlying reality to human being, rather than merely an image with certain attributes. She says,

> To the Father – the primordial creator – from whom everything derives its existence but who himself exists only by and through his own self, would then correspond the being of the soul, while to the Son – the 'born-out' essential form – would correspond all bodily being. And the free and selfless streaming forth (of the Holy Spirit) would have its counterpart in the activity of the spirit, which merits the name spirit [*Geist*] in a special sense.
>
> (Stein, 2002, p. 361)

She goes on to argue that animals have a body-soul unity, but no consciousness of an I which experiences and makes choices. "The animal-ego is more or less at the mercy of 'drives' [*Getriebe*] of its life. It does not stand personally erect [*aufgerichtet*] behind and above them" (Stein, 2002, p. 370). Animals might be understood as having physical and sentient layers, but not mental layers in her descriptions. She immediately goes on to discuss how this is different for the body-soul-spirit unity in human being:

> In the human soul personal erectness has become a fact. Here the inner life has become conscious being. The I has been awakened, and its vision moves in an outward and inward direction. The I is capable of viewing the multitude of external impressions in the light of its understanding and of responding to them in personal freedom [...] People do not, however, make full use of their freedom but rather abandon themselves to a large extent – much in the manner of merely sentient creatures – to the pressures and forces of external and internal 'events' and 'drives' [*Geschehen und Treiben*].
>
> (Stein, 2002, p. 370)

This description resonates with Teresa of Avila's description of the soul as an interior castle, since the 'I' might spend more or less time in the outer mansions of the castle, where it is influenced by external and 'superficial' events and responds to internal drives without full consideration. Having explored how human beings are different from animals, Stein then explains how human beings have less freedom than pure spirits, even though the angels are also limited in freedom since they are not authors of their own being, as God the Father is. She says the angels receive their being/existence as a gift over and over again and, of course, they have no physical body. She argues that the human soul, with a spiritual body, animates the human physical body, and so carries itself within a physical body. Human beings have freedom to make choices about how to act with their bodies, but at times have no control over the reactions of their bodies to physical conditions.

Stein continues to use her belief in the Trinity as an approach to understanding the relationship between body, soul, and spirit, where she suggests there is another three-in-one relationship activated. It is also possible to glimpse another aspect of Stein's method here, as she demonstrates how an exploration of extremes allows her to consider, if humans are 'more' than animals and 'less' than pure spirit, what that might suggest for human being. Her considerations have her posit that human being is born in a similar condition to that of animals, since their bodies and awareness grow in predetermined developmental patterns, but that, at a certain point, human beings also develop an 'I', or consciousness, when it becomes possible for the self to begin observing and reflecting upon itself. Prior to this, children (and animals) may have a sense of themselves receiving and acting in the world but would not consider their 'I' as an object to be studied or understood.

Stein goes on, drawing directly from Teresa of Avila's work,

> The soul as interior castle – as it was pictured by our holy mother Teresa – is not point-like [...], but 'spatial.' It is a space, a 'castle' with many mansions in which the I is able to move freely, now going outward beyond itself, now withdrawing into its own inwardness. And this space is not 'empty,' even though it can and must receive and harbor a fullness in order to become capable of unfolding its own individual life.
>
> (Stein, 2002, p. 373)

This raises more clearly the question of what this sense of self, or 'I', is and how this is different from, or similar to, the soul, which is something Teresa did not explore. Stein answers this question later when she says,

> Ego [or I] and soul are not merely juxtaposed, but inseparably linked. To the human soul there belongs a personal ego that dwells in the soul, that embraces the soul, and in whose life the being of the soul becomes a living and conscious presence. And the human ego is so constituted that its life rises out of the dark depth of the soul.
>
> (Stein, 2002, p. 431)

In describing the journey of the I, gaining ever more complex levels of self-knowledge, Stein not only uses Teresa's image of inner mansions of a castle, she also uses the image of going below the surface of a body of water. She argues that the I, or the awakened sense of self that can reflect upon itself, is the entrance way to the hidden life of the soul, although experiences in the soul may occur at lesser/outer or deeper/inner realms. The I can begin to study the soul as an object even though the I and the soul are closely related. Just as Teresa points out, intellect and self-knowledge are only going to assist with this study of the soul, or journey to the inner mansions, so far. Stein argues that there is a certain type of understanding that can strike more deeply than just the intellect, engaging the whole human being/the whole soul in such a way that even "bodily organs, the heartbeat, and the rhythm of breathing, the individual's sleep and digestion" are all affected (Stein, 2002, p. 437). She goes on to say that the soul takes part in a call and response process, where something may motivate the person to act in a certain way, to make a stand, or to take a position based on the meaning made of a particular context (p. 439). (This language is consistent with the language of narrative therapy theory and practice, which I will return to in chapter eight.) Stein goes on to say,

> The personal I is most truly at home in the innermost being of the soul. When the I loves its life in this interiority, it is then capable of freely disposing of and of freely engaging the soul's collected power. In this interiority the I is also closest to the meaning of every event, most open to the demands with which it is confronted, and in the best possible position to evaluate the significance and the import of these demands. Few human beings, however, live such 'collected' lives. The ego of most of them takes a stand on the surface.
>
> (Stein, 2002, p. 439)

Stein also suggests that during the course of a human being's life, prior to consciousness of the possible depths of the soul, the soul will have been affected by past decisions and behaviours and so will have developed coverings which need to be broken through. These initial mansions, or shallow depths, do not involve "the true interiority of the soul, but merely the residue of the original life of the soul, or those crusts which, steadily growing, cover and hide the inner life of the soul" (Stein, 2002, p. 443).

Returning to the concepts of potency (potential) and act, Stein argues that human being has a passive form of potency, since free will is involved and the potential to act is not always engaged. However, she also suggests,

> The spiritual nature [*Geistnatur*] of the soul is presupposed for its union with God (i.e., for its life of grace and glory). In this union the soul ascends to a height of being that places it side by side with pure spirits. But the soul is distinguished from pure spirits in that the union (the life of grace and glory) is in the case of the soul an 'ascent' or 'an elevation.' For the being of pure spirits consists in the most real sense in their free self-surrender to God and his service – the only alternative possibility being the refusal of self-surrender on the part of evil spirits. The soul, on the other hand, has to fulfill a double (or triple) task. It has to form itself by unfolding its own essence or nature; it has to form or inform the body; and it is to ascend above itself to union with God.
>
> (Stein, 2002, pp. 459–460)

In this way, drawing upon the image of St. John of the Cross's *Ascent to Mount Carmel*, (pp. 436–444), Stein is describing human being's potential, as well as the work, or acts, required to unleash that potential. The soul works to develop itself and form the material body, but it also has the opportunity, through an ever-deepening or inner journey, to become more than that through a relationship with the Divine. This inner journey may involve a sense of 'darkness' or 'nothingness' as one stage of this unfolding.

The Night-symbol and Nothingness in Unfolding

In *SC*, Stein quotes John of the Cross as saying, "Only when the soul is reduced to nothing, the highest degree of humility, will the spiritual union [...] with God be an accomplished fact" (2018, p. 32). Having stated that God has created human souls for himself and that he desires to unite them to himself so that they may experience a fullness of life, she presents an exploration of John's use of 'cross' and 'night' as two different types of symbols in this process of journeying toward spiritual union. Although the 'cross' can be considered a human-made object which acts as an 'emblem' due to the manner in which it has gained meaning over time, she suggests 'night' is something natural, which is not an object but rather something invisible and formless which wraps itself around us. Although light reveals visible qualities, she says night devours them, which can at times seem frightening, but she goes on to describe the loveliness of twilight and moonlight, suggesting it is easier in twilight to hear voices that might otherwise be drowned out in bright daylight. She suggests that comparing "cosmic night" to "mystical night" provides a relationship of "symbolic expression" (p. 41), and a way to understand the movement from meditation (which involves the intellect) through contemplation (which detaches itself from intellect) toward union with God. This could also be described as a process of an essence and its potential "unfolding"; although Stein only briefly uses this term in *FEB*, Gricoski (2020) has recently explored her use of it, and I will touch upon it also in relation to the growth that can come about through the three stages of the mystical night. One challenge with these images of stages and of unfolding and growth is that they can imply a deterministic and linear process, whereas it may be more useful to think of the overall spiritual journey as more cyclical in nature.

This mystical symbol of 'night' and the feeling of 'nothingness' in the darkest stage of the night may offer one way of understanding a person's therapeutic journey through despair and toward wholeness. This therapeutic journey could also be described as a form of unfolding into possibilities, or, to use Stein's terms, an unfolding of potency into action. I will, therefore, ground my discussion of 'night' and 'nothingness' within another case example from my psychotherapeutic practice. Of course, not everyone who engages in psychotherapy is necessarily interested in deepening a relationship with God, but as Rohr suggests,

> After years of counseling both religious and nonreligious people, it seems to me that most humans need a love object. [...] Love grounds

> us by creating focus, direction, motivation, even joy [...] In some ways, the object of our affection is arbitrary. It can begin as a love of golf, a clean house, your cat, or a desire to cultivate a certain reputation for yourself. Granted, the largeness of the object will eventually determine the largeness of the love, but God will use anything to get us started, focused, and flowing. Only a very few actually start this journey with God as the object. [...] God is clearly humble and does not seem to care who or what gets the credit. Whatever elicits the flow for you – in that moment and encounter, that thing is God for you! I do not say that without theological foundation, because my Trinitarian faith says that God is Relationship Itself. The names of the three "persons" of the Trinity are not as important as the relationship between them. That's where all the power is – in the "in between"!
> (https://cac.org/love-is-life-giving-2021-03-16/)

With these ideas of 'anything getting us started' and the importance of the 'in between' in mind, I will describe Emma,[2] who said she was not religious, but who also suggested the search for love was confusing and unsettling her, leading her into what appeared to be a liminal, or betwixt and between place. In speaking with the intake worker, Emma merely stated that she wished to discuss issues from her past which were causing her some anxiety. Her case was assigned to me and in my first appointment with her (online with video connection, due to COVID-19 restrictions), I asked her about her preferred pronouns and whether, when she mentioned a relationship that was ending, she was referring to a same-sex or heterosexual relationship. She looked shocked to be asked and said, 'It's funny you should ask, because that is what I want to talk about'. In the next few appointments, Emma went on to talk about a history of childhood trauma, a growing sense of being attracted to other women and wanting to have a same-sex relationship. She spoke about the fear of coming out to family members and friends and cried for much of our meetings as she described her sense of confusion, sadness, and fear.

Although I have been a psychotherapist for 30 years, with much of that time involving full-time work in a counseling agency where I provided counseling to adult survivors of childhood sexual abuse, and people who had been victimized by, or who had perpetrated, intimate partner violence, there was something about the manner in which Emma presented her situation that I found particularly impactful. As a narrative therapist, I do not usually reflect upon the role of psychodynamic concepts of transference and counter-transference in my work, but my reactions to Emma had me thinking about whether I was engaged in a process of counter-transference as I felt I was perhaps overreacting, and wanting to save her from her sense of despair in a way I hadn't reacted in other traumatic case situations. There was something that seemed to suggest she was struggling with a sense of nothing being secure and a sense of feeling close to the end of her rope. She reported being able to go through the motions of self-care, going for walks in nature, and trying to do some journaling at times, but otherwise she described feeling totally alone and that she would never be happy because she said she felt she had left it too late in life as a 40-year-old to question her sexuality and make a new lifestyle. I will come back to Emma, as I discuss some of my considerations when working with her.

Postmodern and Traditional Psychotherapeutic Understandings of the Liminal Space

As I have indicated in previous chapters, I have found it particularly useful to use the structures of conversational maps that White (2007) developed in my therapeutic practice; influenced by Russian developmental psychologist, Lev Vygotsky, White has described this movement from the "known and familiar" as going through "zones of proximal development" as we attempt to scaffold the conversation in such a way that the person does not experience a sense of not-knowing, but of guided explorations of things known toward the "possible to know". White was also influenced by French ethnographer, Arnold van Gennep, and his work on rites passage, further describing the process of counseling as moving from a particular place or way of being, through a liminal, or betwixt and between stage, and on toward a new location or identity. Describing this passage as a migration of identity within the therapeutic context, this setting forth from what is familiar, into the unknown, even if with some particular goal in mind, can be exceptionally unsettling for people at times. This has always made sense to me since it has described much of what I have witnessed in therapeutic settings, but the fear and uncertainty within this liminal space appeared to be all the more intense for Emma, as described above. I felt out of step with her at times, as I took up a lesbian-affirming position with her, but she had not yet taken up a lesbian-affirming position herself, as she continued to question her sexuality.

Lawver (2012) describes his struggles with a similar case, and not wanting to be drawn into a debate regarding her questioning of her sexuality, focused on his patient's story of trauma. I attempted to work this way with Emma, which provided her space and time to reconsider her relationship to her childhood, yet she soon focused back on her sadness related to her questioning of her sexuality and her fear of coming out. I slipped into providing information more than I usually would and started worrying about whether I was going to be helpful or not, although I also assisted her in developing some grounding techniques to manage her anxiety and rumination. Oddly, it took several weeks for me to realize Emma's situation was perhaps involving fear and discomfort with the liminal stage of counseling and a sense of the 'void' she was experiencing as she contemplated letting go of one identity as she leant toward another. Indeed, I am suggesting this liminal stage in the therapeutic or change process can be experienced as a sense of nothingness and darkness.

Emanuel (2001) writes as a psychoanalytic child and adult psychotherapist, describing his work with people who have had experience with a sense of an overwhelming void, or nothingness, and who then attempt to 'a-void' that experience through particular defense mechanisms. He begins by saying this void is like the experience of the possibility of non-existence and similar to "descriptions of the infant's primitive anxieties of falling to pieces, disintegrating or liquefying, or dropping into the void itself, a terror-inducing, nowhere place, object or space, full of 'nameless dread'" (Emanuel, 2001, p. 1069). He says some people develop sleeping difficulties, separation anxiety, or boredom and anxiety as two sides of the same coin. He says others manage by becoming overly busy and distracting themselves, or by searching for a "known and fixed sense of identity" (p. 1073). However, moving on to integrate a Buddhist perspective with psychoanalytic thought, he states, "there is no such thing as a stable sense of self or true self" (p. 1077).

Emanuel concludes by saying infantile transference is rare in the person who is "a-voiding" since the person "feels remote and inaccessible in the usual sense" (2001, p. 1080). Due to this, he says it is more productive to describe the world the person is living in, sharing your own thoughts and feelings, as the therapist, in order to attempt to reach the other. In doing this, he suggests, we are trying to name the dread and "encourage a kind of courageous mindfulness to attend to the present and the potential in it for growth and change" (p. 1080). He then quotes Eigen, who says:

> What is crucial is how one relates to whatever one may be relating to [...] If, for example, one's emotional reality or truth is despair, what is most important is not that one may be in despair, but one's attitude towards one's despair. Through one's basic attentiveness one's despair can declare itself and tell its story. One enters profound dialogue with it. If one stays with this process an evolution even in the quality of the despair may begin to be perceived, since despair itself is never uniform.
> (Eigen in Emanuel, 2001, p. 1080)

This idea that what is most important is a person's attitude toward the despair circles me back to narrative practices and the idea of considering the "absent but implicit" in what people say in therapeutic conversations (Béres, 2014; Carey, Walther, & Russell, 2009; White, 2007). This idea that people's knowledge, skills, and values are often not explicitly articulated but rather only implied, is also related to the importance of asking people about how certain feelings or thoughts have changed over time; asking, for instance, about how despair may have been less or more at different times. This practice demonstrates the therapist's curiosity regarding how the liminal stage is changing over time, assuming the despair and darkness will not always be experienced in exactly the same way. Relating this to Edith Stein's explorations, this is like bringing attention to the manner in which cosmic night is made up of different periods, beginning with twilight, and how these elements of the symbol of night might assist us in understanding mystical night in more detail.

In describing John of the Cross's work in *SC*, Stein uses the term 'detachment' to describe some of what the soul needs to experience, which, as I have suggested in the previous chapters, shares some elements in common with the Buddhist concept of 'non-attachment' and 'no-self'. She says,

> Detachment is designated as a night through which the soul must pass. It is this in a threefold sense: in regard to the point of departure, the path, and the goal. The point of departure is the desire for the things of this world, which the soul must renounce. But this renunciation transplants her into darkness and as though into nothingness. That is why it is called night.
>
> (Stein, 2018, pp. 45–46)

She describes this night symbol as sharing similarities with the 'real-world' night, or cosmic night as she calls it. She says the cosmic night, from twilight, through the darkest hours, and on to dawn, is not equally dark throughout, and so the mystic night also has different times and intensities. She says,

> The submersion of the world of the senses is like the oncoming of night, when a mere twilight remains of the day's brightness. Faith, on the contrary, is the midnight darkness because here not only are the senses inactive but the knowledge from natural understanding is eliminated. The dawn of the new day of eternity, however, breaks into her night when the soul finds God.
>
> (Stein, 2018, p. 46)

As Tyler (2010) comments, John of the Cross was writing in the south of Spain, and so those of us living in cooler, damper regions of the world, might want to remember that John's night would have been like a "warm silky Spanish night of high summer full of delicate scents, murmuring sounds, strange birds, moths and insects and the light breeze" (p. 8). This reminder is consistent with Stein's comments regarding the beauty of twilight. However, she also relates this journey through stages of the night, in a manner that appears similar to the idea of outer and inner mansions of the soul, with corresponding differences in focus and reliance on the intellect; indeed, she says the more we withdraw from the sensory (the outer experiences) the more the spiritual and inner aspects of our souls arise (Stein, 2018, p. 55). She reiterates that the intellect, by its own power, only takes us so far (p. 58).

This three-stage description of the cosmic and mystical night is similar to van Gennep's description of "rites of passage" (usually involving a ritual of some sort) which has influenced the idea of the "migration of identity" in narrative practices described above; people leave a familiar territory and set sail into the unknown with only a sense of where they may land. Despite the beauty of the twilight element of night, the darkest stage of night requires faith. Stein has suggested that through the process of recognizing the intellect cannot help, and then experiencing a period of confusion and trials, the soul becomes humble (which was important to Teresa of Avila also), resulting in a sense of peace, patience, and courage. She suggests that not all people are tested in the same degree, but that "[t]he higher degree of union of love to which God desires to lead them, the more intense and prolonged will the purification be" (p. 54). Those in therapy, without faith, might experience 'dark' times like these, although not initiated by prayer and mindfulness, as particularly frightening.

The Darkest Stage of the Night

Regarding the darkest stage of the night process, Stein says,

> [I]t has not only been made clear that faith is a dark night, but also that it is a way: the way to the goal toward which the soul strives, to union with God. For it alone gives knowledge of God. And how is one to arrive at union with God without knowing him? [...] She must enter into the night of faith of her own choice and by her own power. [...] she must now die to her natural faculties, her senses, and to her intellect also. For in order to reach the supernatural transformation, she must leave behind everything natural.
>
> (Stein, 2018, p. 59)

She adds that this process involves simply believing in God's existence which is not founded on any sort of intellect, will, or imagination, pointing out that, "in order to attain to God, one must "rather strive [...] *not* [italics added] to understand as to understand ... rather to be blind and transport oneself into darkness [...] than to open the eyes" (p. 66). She then goes on to present how John of the Cross describes the types of knowledge, and the manner in which these knowledges come to a person, during this darkest part of the night. Although John distinguishes spiritual communications as being experienced as "spiritual visions, revelations, locations, and feelings" (p. 71), and although Stein reviews the differences between each of these forms of communication, she is also clear that it is important to also discuss these experiences with a trusted spiritual director due to the possibility of misunderstanding. She warns that a soul may begin to believe she has experienced something great and in so doing allow herself to be distracted from "the abyss of faith" (p. 76).

Although the focus is different within spiritual direction as opposed to psychotherapy, this idea of checking with a spiritual director sounds similar to checking in with a therapist. As a person experiences the darkest period of night, or a sense of this abyss, whether brought about due to meditation, contemplation, and a desire to experience the Divine, or due to external or internal experiences of questioning themselves, their identity and feeling in a betwixt and between place, checking in with a trusted counselor along the journey can be useful. After all, it can be frightening, to come to the point in this process when neither the will, nor the intellect, can assist with planning for next steps. As O'Donohue points out, which is reminiscent of Lydia's experience described in the last chapter,

> Too often people try to change their lives by using the will as a kind of hammer to beat their life into proper shape. The intellect identifies the goal of the program, and the will accordingly forces the life into that shape. This way of approaching sacredness of one's own presence is externalist and violent. […] If you work with a different rhythm, you will come easily and naturally home to yourself. Your soul knows the geography of your destiny. Your soul alone has the map of your future, therefore you can trust this indirect, oblique side of yourself. If you do, it will take you where you need to go, but more importantly, it will teach you a kindness of rhythm in your journey.
>
> (O'Donohue, 1997, pp. 57–80)

If someone has relied on their intellect and their will in all that they have accomplished to this point, realizing that their usual approach will no longer work can be both humbling and frightening, but also can lead to much more satisfying outcomes if they are willing to surrender to this sense of nothingness. Another image for the process of change that can occur through surrendering to nothingness is that of unfolding.

Unfolding toward the Third Stage of Night: Dawn

Gricoski has focused on Stein's later Christian, and more metaphysical, work and specifically her comments on "unfolding" in *FEB*, which she first explored through her interest in human being's potential in *PA*. Gricoski says, "The principle of 'unfolding' holds meaning and being in irreducible relationship in all types of finite being. 'Meaning' refers to the essence of individual things including all of their potentialities as well as universals" (2020, p. xviii). He goes on to explain he is using a relational ontology, by which he means "a theory of being which places relationships at the ground level of metaphysics" (p. xviii) and then points out that "unfolding" is a relational principle, where "unfolding is the unfolding of something else" (p. xix). He suggests Stein was influenced by her friend and colleague, Hedwig Conrad-Martius, and her philosophical ruminations on plant life, where plants "unfold" themselves over time. He then goes on to describe the phenomenological process of philosophical reflection, relying on a suspension of beliefs, and shifting of viewpoints. He provides the example of Stein looking at a cherry tree in bloom in the Carmelite cloisters in Cologne. He suggests she initially views the tree simply as it appears to her – a beautiful cherry tree, covered in blossoms. However, she then moves into the position of phenomenologist and philosopher, aware that categories which she understands are used to make judgments about her perceptions. She needs to bracket these categories to attempt to engage with the essence of the tree:

> In order to intuit the essence of the tree, the philosopher imaginatively varies the tree's features. Imagine that the tree is a meter taller; it remains a cherry tree. Imagine going back in time to when it was a seedling sprouting from the ground; the essence of the tree remains the same. Try to imagine the tree spouting peaches, and one finds that the essence of the cherry tree resists this variation. The object of these latter intentions is no longer the essence of a cherry tree.
>
> (Gricoski, 2020, p. 14)

This description of reflecting upon the cherry tree, and another example Gricoski presents in relation to considering lumps of gold compared to an ideal image of gold, are helpful as he moves on to describe Stein's account of humans unfolding. He says that no finite object exists without gesturing toward something beyond itself.

> The ideal, or rather, the essential, to which earthly imperfections point, however, is not a "perfect earth" or an ideal utopia. These images of utopian perfection are also deficient compared to the essential sphere. A world inhabited by perfect persons living among perfect plants and animals would still be irremediably "deficient". The constant comparison is not simply between actual finite beings and ideal finite beings, but more so between finite being and the perfect eternal being.
>
> (Gricoski, 2020, p. 225)

Stein does not blame finite objects for this, but rather says,

> It lies in the meaning of creation that the created cannot be a perfect likeness [*vollkommenes Abbild*], but only a "partial likeness" [*Teilbild*], a "broken ray". God, the eternal, uncreated and infinite, cannot create an equal, because there cannot be a second eternal, uncreated and infinite [being].
>
> (Stein in Gricoski, 2020, p. 235)

I have found these reflections on unfolding helpful as a further analogy for considering the journey through the three stages of cosmic and mystical night, including the darkest stage that is like a void where nothing can be relied upon other than faith. Indeed, Stein argues in *SC*, "In faith the spirit is painfully reborn; it is remodeled from the natural to the supernatural. [...] For insofar as spiritual being is life and change, it cannot be captured in static definitions, but must rather be a continual movement seeking fluid expression" (2018, p. 112). Stein suggests that the soul "is buried in corporeality and has senses which are bound to the body as receptive organs for whatever is material" (p. 118), and even those people who are committed to daily contemplative prayer and meditation continue to have "both feet firmly planted on the ground" (p. 119). However, as has been described above, people can only travel so far with their own skills and intellect and must detach themselves even from all that seems spiritually good.

As she continues to explore John of the Cross's reflections, Stein describes the dark night as purging imperfections from the soul in order to enkindle love, transformation, and preparation for union with God (2018, p. 133). At this point the image of being set aglow by fire is used. During this process the soul is weaned from its natural appetites and undergoes "a cure to regain her health" (p. 139). Stein explores John's imagery of the "secret ladder" and the manner in which a soul can ascend and descend this ladder, while also using depth metaphors and those from Teresa of Avila's interior castle, with inner and outer layers of mansions. She then proceeds to argue that a soul has an experience of an I which can ascend or descend that ladder and move between greater or lesser depths or inner and outer mansions. She says the I moves about due to her own motivations and will depending on her preferences, but once she has chosen to allow herself to be drawn to that innermost place where God otherwise lives alone, she then reaches perfect union. She says, "the autonomous action of the soul apparently diminishes the more she nears her inmost self. And when she arrives there, God does everything in her, she no longer has anything more to do than receive. However, it is precisely this act of receiving that expresses her free participation. [...] God does everything here only because the soul has totally surrendered herself to him. And this surrender is the highest act of freedom" (p. 162). Nonetheless, she says something is still missing.

Stein explains John of the Cross distinguishes three types of union with God. The first is in regard to God dwelling in and sustaining the existence of all created things. The second is related to God's dwelling in the soul through grace, and the third relates to "the transforming union through perfect love that divinizes the soul" (p. 167). These second and third forms of union are described as corresponding to each other like "betrothal and marriage" (p. 172) while Stein points out that Teresa of Avila and John of the Cross could not write about these experiences completely clearly, always having to reckon with the Inquisition and the risk of charges of heresy (as described in the last chapter). However, John has also written of how, once the soul has traveled through the night, there is a sense of being bathed in the brilliance of the "Resurrection morning" (p. 187). Stein points out, though, that the delight and experience of this is still not happening here as perfectly as it will in eternal life – which resonates with Gricoski's reminders above about the difference between 'perfect in this world' and 'the perfect divine image'. Despite this, further images are called upon that suggest the great changes in love and faith that can come about due to the movement from twilight, through 'nothingness' in the darkest stage of night, and into the dawn of a new day, suggesting these changes are like that of a caterpillar becoming a butterfly, or a mustard seed becoming a large mustard tree. Of course, there is, conceivably, a corresponding darkness within the chrysalis before the butterfly emerges, and within the soil as the seed gestates.

Conclusion

Stein's conceptions and language of the soul, I believe, are consistent with, but also add to the language of postmodern therapies. For instance, for her, the human being is not a closed system, nor is it as simple as taught in much of psychology. As Sawicki (2000) suggests, Stein would have found many of today's psychological theories far too narrowly focused. Stein, rather, was fascinated by those times when people manage what would seem unpredictable and accomplish more than they could even have imagined themselves capable, like moving from a problem storyline to a preferred storyline. Using a phenomenological approach has allowed her to present a description of the complexity of human being.

After Stein's conversion, as she incorporated her Christian faith into her work, her explorations regarding the layers of human being were further enriched, as she also added Aquinas's scholastic approach. People can still be seen to be living in the surfaces of their being, socially constructing their identities through the stories they tell about themselves, as narrative therapists would suggest. However, when and if they begin to explore those inner aspects, or depths of themselves, moving beyond even just 'self-knowledge' to those realms of mystery and possibility, she (and Teresa of Avila) provide possible road maps and suggestions for how to understand and potentially support the deepening of these experiences.

In this chapter, I have also drawn upon Stein's reflections on the images of 'cosmic night' and the 'nothingness' associated with the darkest part of the night. The fact that twilight eases into darkness and that dawn rises gently adds a certain degree of gentleness and comfort. John of the Cross and Stein have admitted there can be discomfort in the darkest stage of the night, but once the joy of union with the Divine has been experienced, the soul does not fear these discomforts. Stein explains these moments of union are short-lived for finite beings in a finite world, and so this three-stage process is not a one-time event, but rather a process that can occur time and again.

Regarding my work with Emma, she also has come through her darkest stage of her therapeutic process and is seeing glimmers of light as she has begun a new relationship – with a woman. She told me that she has also started the process of 'coming out' to friends and family, having had a good experience with this so far and looking forward to telling more people. She says she is feeling more authentically her real self now than ever before, but she may, of course, experience liminal and betwixt and between times again.

While the notion of our true essence unfolding on this journey through night has also been useful, I wonder whether the image of a flower opening and closing depending on the amount of light present might also correspond to our journeys, since we are not always in a state of union with the Divine. Our 'I' moves in and out of various levels of our soul, and is more preoccupied with the world at times, and more at rest with God at other times. Since no symbol is perfect for the analogy of the journey to wholeness, this image of light and dark is also not perfect and requires a shift when considering the flower unfolding in God's light, which occurs in the inner mansion of the soul, which has previously corresponded to the darkest stage of the night. Thus, we have another example of the need to let go of categories, intellect, and symbols, in order to experience 'nothingness' which has so fascinated the mystics such as Terresa of Avila, John of the Cross, and Edith Stein.

Notes

1 An earlier, shorter, version of this chapter was published in a collection of papers which were presented at the 5th *Biannual International Conference of the International Association for the Study of the Philosophy of Edith Stein*: Béres, L. (2021). Edith Stein's contributions to understandings about the soul for postmodern therapeutic practices. In H. Klueting & E Kuleting (Eds). *Edith Stein's Itinerary: Phenomenology, Christian Philosophy, and Carmelite Spirituality* (pp. 641–650). Aschendorff Verlag. I am grateful for the publisher's permission to re-use this material here.

2 All names and identifying details of clients and case examples have been changed throughout this book.

References

Béres, L. (2014). *The narrative practitioner.* Palgrave MacMillan.

Borden, S. (2003). *Edith Stein.* Continuum.

Calcagno, A. (2007). *The philosophy of Edith Stein.* Duquesne University Press.

Carey, M., Walther, S., & Russell, S. (2009). The absent but implicit: A map to support therapeutic inquiry, *Family Process, 48*(3), 319–331.

Emanuel, R. (2001). A-void – an exploration of defenses against sensing nothingness. *Int. J Psychoanal, 82*, 1069–1084.

Gelber, L. & Leuven, R. (1949). Editors' preface. In *Finite and eternal being: An attempt at an ascent to the meaning of being.* (K. F. Reinhardt, Trans.) (pp. xxiii–xxv). ICS Publications.

Gilson, E. (1952). *Being and some philosophers (2nd. ed.).* Pontifical Institute of Medieval Studies.

Gricoski, T. (2020). *Being unfolded: Edith Stein on the meaning of being*. The Catholic University of America Press.

Lawver, T. I. (2012). Sexuality as focus of therapy: A case study in attribution. *Journal of Gay & Lesbian Mental Health, 16*(1), 66–73. DOI: 10.1080/19359705.2010.551040

McInerny, R. & O'Callaghan, J. (Winter 2016). Saint Thomas Aquinas. *The Stanford encyclopedia of philosophy*. Zalta, E. N., (Ed.). Available at https://plato.standford.edu/archives/win2016/entries/aquinas/. Accessed 21 January 2017.

O'Donohue, J. (1997). *Anam cara: A book of Celtic wisdom*. Cliff Street Books, an imprint of Harper Collins Publishers.

Payne, S. (2000). Preface to the ICS Publications Edition. In M. Sawicki (Ed.). (M. C. Baseheart and M. Sawicki, Trans.). *Philosophy of psychology and the humanities* (pp. IX–X). ICS Publications.

Sawicki, M. (2000). Editor's Introduction. In M. Sawicki (Ed.). (M. C. Baseheart and M. Sawicki, Trans.). *Philosophy of psychology and the humanities* (pp. XI–XXIII). ICS Publications.

Stein. E. (2000). *Philosophy of psychology and the humanities*. M. Sawicki (Ed.). (M. C. Baseheart and M. Sawicki, Trans.) ICS Publications. (Original work published in 1922.)

Stein, E. (2002). *Finite and eternal being: An attempt at an ascent to the meaning of being*. (K. F. Reinhardt, Trans.) ICS Publications. (Original work published in 1949.)

Stein, E. (2009). *Potency and act*. (W. Redmond, Trans.) ICS Publications. (Original work published in 1998.)

Stein, E. (2018). *The Science of the Cross*. (J. Koeppel, O.C.D., Trans.) ICS Publications. (Original work published in 1983.)

Tyler, P. (2010). *St. John of the Cross*. Continuum.

Tyler, P. (2016). *The pursuit of the soul: Psychoanalysis, soul-making and the Christian tradition*. Bloomsbury T & T Clark.

White, M. (2007). *Maps of narrative practice*. W.W. Norton.

6 The *Embodied* Soul: Considering Merleau-Ponty's Contributions to the Language of the Soul

Laura Béres

I recently presented at an online conference regarding a research project in which colleagues and I are examining the links between spirituality and resilience during the COVID-19 pandemic. We focused our presentation on themes found within the first round of transcribed interviews; one of those themes came from findings that showed a link between the body and spirituality, as research participants explained some of their spiritual practices that were assisting them with coping with the pandemic which involved their body as they walked in nature, or purposefully slowed their breath in mindfulness practices, took time to 'step away' from their work 3–6 times each day, or reflected upon their place in physical spaces related to other bodies. These findings were of particular interest to those who attended our conference presentation who work in the medical field and so treat people's bodies, and also to those who have their own embodied spiritual practices such as yoga. Indeed, ensuring that discussions about spirituality and the soul do not become too ethereal, disembodied, and separated from the rest of the physical world is also important for those of us providing psychotherapy, pastoral counseling, and spiritual direction. We are interacting with embodied people in the physical world, and although the soul may have been missing recently from much of the literature about therapeutic practices, in reintroducing the language of the soul to these practices it is important that the pendulum not swing so far in the opposite direction that the importance of the body is lessened; we perhaps should focus on considering the *embodied* soul.

As has been described in the last two chapters, Teresa of Avila and Edith Stein both consider the soul as multilayered, or multifaceted, and as including the physical body, thus moving away from the dualism of body and soul. They have both described how the 'I' (sense of conscious self) can move about within various aspects of the soul, including the outer layers of the soul – the body – as it interacts with the rest of the physical world, and yet can also move into the inner areas of the soul that feel far removed from the world. In the last chapter, I presented Stein's descriptions of the soul, as she suggests, "The soul […] has to fulfill a double (or triple) task. It has to

DOI: 10.4324/9781003137450-9

form itself by unfolding its own essence or nature; it has to *form or inform the body* [italics added]; and it is to ascend above itself to union with [the Divine]" (Stein, 2002, p. 460). She also describes the soul as "buried in corporeality and [having] senses which are bound to the body as receptive organs for whatever is material" (2018, p. 118), and so even those people who are committed to daily contemplative prayer and meditation continue to have "both feet firmly planted on the ground" (p. 119). Idealists and neo-Kantian philosophers suggest that everything we experience is a result of our mind/spirit, and phenomenologists, such as Husserl and Stein, argue that we need to consider *both* consciousness (the mind, or the subject as the witness of an experience) *and* the object (that which is observed by that consciousness/subject) to truly understand an experience/phenomenon. Since this can unfortunately imply a stark separation between mind and matter, Merleau-Ponty attempts to straddle this difference by building upon Husserl's phenomenology as he provides a description of the manner in which the body is integral to perception – a meeting place for mind-world engagement.

In order to provide a practice context within which to consider Merleau-Ponty's contributions to explorations regarding the link between the body and soul, I will present a brief case example of my counseling experience with a young trans woman, named Eve.[1] It may seem particularly important to consider the role of the body for someone who decides to pursue surgery in order to facilitate a greater comfort with their identity and gendered place in the world, but considering the body as part of the perception of experience can be useful for all our practices. Merleau-Ponty, in fact, would more specifically suggest the body is integral to having experiences at all. Although Eve did not request counseling to support her transitioning, this experience was clearly of fundamental importance to her. She requested counseling to assist her with managing anxiety, particularly in relation to the pandemic but also wished to explore the impacts of earlier experiences in her life. In response to my initial queries, she indicated preferring the pronouns 'she/her' and stated she was married to a person who preferred the pronouns 'they/their'. Within a later session, she also explained that she and her partner had an open relationship and she maintained other intimate relationships although she also described herself as ace, or asexual. Interestingly – and consistent with a strengths-focus and interest in preferred storylines within narrative practices – she explained that she prefers to talk in terms of 'euphoria' rather than 'body dysphoria', going on to say that from the time she was a young child she felt better in dresses and skirts than she did dressing in traditional masculine ways. At the age of 20 she was able to have bottom surgery and she has been actively focused on maintaining these surgical changes, developing ever greater levels of comfort with herself and her place in the world. She identifies having a supportive network of friends and good relationships with most of her biological relatives, but still looking for meaningful work/engagement with the world.

Clearly, transitioning from a body that was experienced as out of step with her sense of herself to a body that feels more consistent with herself assists her also in presenting herself more authentically to the rest of the world, easing interactions with others and her resulting perceptions of the world. When asked about whether she would describe herself as having any form of spirituality, she said that she would although it was 'highly personalized and individualized'. For her, as for many spiritual people, spirituality involves a journey toward authenticity and a wish to trust her intuitions. She indicated that she did not particularly resonate with the language of the soul but suggested she was comfortable with the idea of her true Self. The image of the embodied soul as an interior castle with many mansions was not an image I shared with her but it remained in my mind as I interacted with her as a multifaceted embodied soul/Self. Her feedback to me in our final session was that she had felt comfortable with me and supported throughout the counseling process, which she said had not always been true in previous counseling relationships. We laughed about this having been possible despite my identity as a middle-aged white heterosexual cis-gendered woman. In other words, although I did not say this to Eve, I believe it is important to point out that an interest in, and respect for, the soul is not linked to any collusion with fundamentalist religions which are often opposed to 2SLGBTQ+ people and their rights and freedoms to be their authentic selves and love whom they choose. If anything, it feels like a 'soulish' practice to be able to support people in moving into ways of being that feel more authentic for them, and this requires consideration of the impact of the body in this process.

In this chapter, I will describe how I was initially introduced to Merleau-Ponty's work on understanding the role of the body in perception and reflection, showing how his ideas are compatible with Teresa of Avila's and Edith Stein's conceptions of human being, and then move on to discuss the implications of his work for an ethic of care for the environment. Although he does not speak in terms of spirituality and sacredness, the manner in which his work has been taken up in relation to the environment resonates with the ancient idea of 'World soul' (*nous*) as described in chapter three, and with Michael White's interest in 'spiritualities of the surface' and his concern for the environment, as described in chapter one.

The usefulness of Merleau-Ponty's work was particularly pointed out to me a few years ago by a former graduate student who was engaged in a Critical Reflection on Practice (CRoP) course I teach each year in the Master of Social Work (MSW) program where I am a faculty member. I have explained the critical reflection process in chapter two so will not repeat it here, but suffice to say, after completing stage one and before moving on to stage two of the process, I asked the MSW students in the CRoP course if they felt anything was missing. Natashia Botelho spoke up and said she thought the body was missing from the CRoP process. Her academic background included an undergraduate degree in psychology and an M.A. in philosophy, with a particular interest in Merleau-Ponty's phenomenology. She was incorporating these previous separate interests into her MSW studies and her practice as a beginning psychotherapist and yoga instructor. I encouraged her to write an article for publication, arguing for the inclusion of the body in CRoP, which she has done (Botelho, 2020); her arguments for an awareness of the impact of the body on our engagement with, and experience of, the world are important, and add further elements to the CRoP process. I am grateful that she heightened my awareness of Merleau-Ponty, who built upon Husserl's phenomenology in a different, but complimentary, manner to Stein, since his work adds further elements to this current project of introducing the language of the soul to narrative therapy, and therapeutic practices more generally.

It has been argued that psychotherapists need to engage with philosophy, and particularly phenomenology, since all psychotherapy practice flows from some sort of belief in human consciousness, meaning, subjectivity, reality, and morality, even if these topics have not been explicitly examined or studied. Hersch believes engagement with these areas through an exploration of what phenomenological philosophy can teach us will be "enormously useful when it comes to understanding the people who come to [us] for help" (2003, p. 5). He believes we need to first consider ontology (the philosophy of being) before moving on to consider epistemology (the philosophy of knowledge) and only later consider issues of validity and finally psychological issues related to helping people psychotherapeutically. He points out the ways in which Descartes's famous reliance on "Cogito" (I think, and the resulting phrase "I think, therefore I am") has had such long-lasting effects in the Western world regarding what we assume about reality and our place in it, without any reflection:

> A central assumption in Cartesian [related to Descartes] epistemology (and Cartesian psychology) is that our primary relationship to Being (i.e., to any external Reality or object) is one of *knowing* an object – that is, of somehow cognitively or rationally grasping it 'within us.' Indeed, the whole of [...] 'representational thinking,' from Descartes to its more recent psychological iterations (e.g., cognitive psychology and the object relations theories of psychoanalysis), rests heavily on such assumptions.
>
> (Hersch, 2003, p. 25)

He worries that psychotherapists are so affected by the "pragmatic-empirical, 'just the facts,' 'how to fix it' culture, we cannot handle questions that have no clear, easy, and precise answers" (p. 29) to the questions raised by philosophy. Yet, he suggests the need for a non-Cartesian starting point, thereby suggesting we engage with the work of modern phenomenological philosophers who have argued against cognitive knowledge as our primary way of engaging with reality. He argues that this means moving away from the implicit assumption of the separation between the subject of consciousness and the object of that consciousness. He provides a description of Husserl's phenomenology, similar to that which I presented in the last chapter as I explained Stein's studies with Husserl, but he particularly draws attention to intentionality within Husserl's work; he clarifies that philosophical intentions are different from psychological intentions (motivations); philosophical intentions have a sense of directedness toward the object of consciousness (p. 48). Although Hersch suggests Husserl never totally overcame dualism in his writing, his valuing of lived experience and the elaboration of the phenomenon of experience in his work makes it very useful for psychotherapists. For narrative therapists, and other psychotherapists, who are particularly interested in "experience-near descriptions" (White, 2007), phenomenologists' exploration of experience is valuable. As stated above, Merleau-Ponty adds the 'lived body' to this analysis of perception or experience.

Merleau-Ponty and Body Phenomenology

Unlike several distinguished philosophers, Maurice Merleau-Ponty (1908–1961) led a life which did not directly affect the essential content and development of his philosophical ideas, although his historical context and experiences no doubt affected his political stance and political writings (Carman, 2020, pp. 6–7). Merleau-Ponty was born and lived most of his life in France. He studied, and later taught and wrote in the areas of existentialism and phenomenology. He studied under Edmund Husserl, was also influenced by Martin Heidegger, and was associated with Jean-Paul Sartre and Simone de Beauvoir although they experienced a falling out over ideological differences. He was also interested in, and attended lectures on, Gestalt psychology, which influenced the development of his form of phenomenology. He then went on to influence Michel Foucault, Gilles Deleuze, and Jacques Derrida. He is best known for *Phenomenology of Perception (PP),* which was published in the original French in 1945. However, his ideas continued to evolve, and his unfinished work was published posthumously as *The Visible and Invisible (VI)* in 1964. (I have read the English translations of these two works.) He was a Professor of Philosophy at the University of Lyon, and later Chair of Philosophy at the Collège de France, yet also spent time as a Professor of Child Psychology and Pedagogy at the Sorbonne University. He was in military service from 1930 to 1931, from 1939 to 1940, and then involved in the Resistance in France until 1944. He died of heart failure at the age of 53 in 1961, shocking his friends and colleagues with his death at such a young age (Carman, 2020; Lefort, 1968).

Carman (2020) suggests there are four main highlights to Merleau-Ponty's work:

1 "[P]erception is not an isolated event or state in the mind or brain but an organism's entire *bodily* relation to its environment. Perception is [...] an 'ecological' phenomenon" (p. 1).
2 "Perception is finite [... and] 'is my point of view on the world'" (p. 1). "I can have a point of view *on* the world only by being *in* the world. I can perceive anything – even my own internal body states like pain or fatigue – only by inhabiting an environment. [...] To see, I must be visible. To touch, I must be tangible" (p. 2).
3 "Confusion about perception persists in part as a natural, perhaps inevitable, effect of a vital tendency at work in perceptual awareness itself, namely our unreflective absorption in the world, our directedness toward objects – hence the systematic deflection of our attention away from our own experience" (p. 2).
4 "Bodily perspective grounds and informs culture, language, art, literature, history, science, and politics. Human conduct in all areas is marked, to a greater or lesser degree, by its bodily aspect, its perspectival orientation, and its inherent tendency toward self-deflection and self-forgetting" (p. 3).

The third point above particularly draws my attention, resonating as it does with the manner in which Teresa of Avila and Edith Stein both describe how humans have a tendency to become caught up and distracted by the world in the outer mansions/layers of their soul. Merleau-Ponty's project involves expanding Husserl's phenomenology to further consider the mind-body-world relationship involved in perception, which involves some of the inner layers of the soul, but specifically involves adding more focus on the environment. This addition of the environment, or context, appears to have been influenced by his interest in Gestalt psychology, and also offers some resonance for social workers trained to consider the "person-in-environment". In addition to, and related to, these four areas of his work which Carman highlights, Merleau-Ponty added the ideas of "flesh" and "chiasm" in his posthumously published *VI*, which I will discuss once I have traced the influence of his earlier work.

Discussing a limitation of classical psychology as being due to psychologists not recognizing that they were unable to *not* be influenced by their own psyches as they ostensibly attempted to objectively study others' psyches, Merleau-Ponty says, "as a psyche speaking of the psyche, [the psychologist] *was* all he [sic] was *talking* about" (Merleau-Ponty, 1978, p. 96). He goes on, using the language of the soul,

> The union of soul and body had not been brought about once and for all in a remote realm, it came into being afresh at every moment beneath the psychologist's thinking, not as a repetitive event which each time takes the psyche by surprise, but as a necessity that the psychologist knew to be in the depths of his being as he became aware

> of it as a piece of knowledge. […], the psychologist's being knew more about itself than he did […] Before being an objective fact, the union of soul and body had to be, then, a possibility of consciousness itself and the question arose as to what the perceiving subject is and whether he must be able to experience a body as his own. […] To be a consciousness or rather *to be an experience* is to hold inner communication with the world, the body and other people, to be with them instead of being beside them.
>
> (Merleau-Ponty, 1978, p. 96)

In this way, Merleau-Ponty is raising questions of how and where the sense of self is engaged in perception within the body soul union. He was interested in the mysteries (versus philosophical problems) of "being, time, truth, knowledge, love, death" (Carman, 2020, p. 7) and in his earlier work was particularly interested in the mystery of perception (p. 8). As Carman (2020) points out, knowing that our retinas receive an image of objects upside down, "[h]ow do we manage to see things right side up and right way around? […] Moreover, most of us have two eyes, not just one, hence two retinal images. Why do we not see double?" (pp. 8–9). There are also the mysteries of how we see hallucinations, and other ideas in our mind's eye. Merleau-Ponty was interested in exploring how and what perception told us of the world, taking into account our point of view in the world – not just intellectually speaking. He was keen to critique rationalism, intellectualism, and cognitivism, which "are all different versions of a common underlying idea, namely that *thought* constitutes our essential relation to the world" (p. 12). His argument was that perception is more basic than thought, since people learn to think about what they first see: "a child perceives before [they] think" (Merleau-Ponty in Carman, 2020, p. 12).

As indicated above, Husserl's phenomenology had an obvious influence on Merleau-Ponty, but especially as I consider the implications of his work for those of us working directly with people in psychotherapy, pastoral counseling, and spiritual direction, it is interesting to also note the impact of Gestalt psychology on Merleau-Ponty's work. Although Gestalt psychology arose in the 1910s and 1920s in Germany, with Max Wertheimer, Kurt Koffka, and Wolfgang Köhler its primary figures, Merleau-Ponty attended lectures on Gestalt psychology from Aron Gurwitsch who was also influenced by reading Husserl's work. (Interestingly, both Husserl's phenomenology and Gestalt psychology developed in Germany.) Gestalt psychology, like narrative therapy, rejects mechanistic assumptions, and, rather, argues that experience has a "holistic and dynamic character in virtue of its intelligible form or shape (Gestalt)" (Carman, 2020, p. 26). A Gestalt, then, is more than a sum of its parts as those various parts are all in relation to one another, within a perceptual field or horizon. For example, in relation to seeing a book on a table, we do not see a range of lines, edges, shapes, and colors and then piece them together, but rather we see "a solid object with a hidden interior and back sides; What [we] see is [...] in this case a solid object in its environment" (Carman, 2020, p. 26). Merleau-Ponty takes up some of this idea of there being hidden interiors to the outer elements of an object that we perceive in *The Visible and the Invisible (VI).*

Carman uses a further clear example to show an additional aspect of Merleau-Ponty's interest in the body's role in perception, as opposed to any tendency to only considering the ways in which our minds intellectually make sense of the world through language and ideas:

> A horse stumbles and catches itself to regain its balance, a cat recoils from a passage it senses is too narrow, a bird cocks its head to hear better the insects in the grass. Like us, more or less sentient and intelligent animals seem to have at least a primitive sense of where they *ought* to be and what they *ought* to do, not, of course, under any linguistically articulate description but simply as somehow optimal or suboptimal, better or worse. This idea, [...] that ordinary perception and behaviour are always organized around a normative notion of rightness or equilibrium is a crucially important insight at work in Merleau-Ponty's phenomenology.
>
> (Carman, 2020, p. 28)

In some ways, this description is consistent with Stein's conception of the physical and sentient layers of a human being, as a human is affected by physical aspects of the environment and can automatically, without thought, adjust to maintain balance while walking on a rocking boat or train, for instance, or cringe as someone else hurts themselves, as described in the last chapter. Describing consciousness, Merleau-Ponty says that it "invades the body, the soul spreads across all of its parts, behaviour overflows its central region" (Merleau-Ponty in Carman, 2020, p. 87). In fact, Merleau-Ponty, like Stein, also considers layers of the person and some types of consciousness as involving an "I":

> Only some of our experience centers around a self-conscious subject, a locus of personal identity and responsibility – in short, an I. Underlying that (more or less) transparent personal subject is a more primitive, one might say merely *translucent* layer of bodily experience that has a more impersonal character better captured by the French pronoun *on* ("one" or "we"), as in *one blinks every few seconds*, or *we breathe through our noses*. The *pre*personal bodily subject of perception is thus not my conscious, reflective self, but simply 'the one' (*le* "*on*").
>
> (Carman, 2020, p. 90)

Merleau-Ponty suggests that it is much more accurate to say 'one sees a blue sky' rather than 'I see a blue sky', since the experience is of a bodily perception of a blue sky rather than a reflecting 'I' that chooses to see the blue sky. There is much more that could be said about this and Merleau-Ponty's descriptions about the role of the body in perception and the challenges associated with the body attempting to observe itself, but I will move on to describe how Merleau-Ponty's interest in perception and embodiment changed in the 1950s.

Carman describes Merleau-Ponty's new direction in his thinking as involving a paradigm shift, similar to that which can be noted in Heidegger's and Wittgenstein's work. His new line of thought is particularly presented in chapter four of *VI,* where he describes 'flesh' and 'chiasm'. Carman describes Merleau-Ponty as abandoning the primacy of consciousness, and rather focusing even more purposefully upon the body's unconscious bodily perceptions, which was influenced by his consideration of the impacts of catastrophic brain damage (2020, p. 115). What is new is how Merleau-Ponty describes the unconscious ground of conscious experience, or ontological bedrock:

> The underlying ontological foundation of sensory receptivity and motor spontaneity is what Merleau-Ponty now calls flesh (*chair* [the French word for 'flesh']). Flesh is the stuff common to ourselves and the world, what we and it are both made of, as it were. And yet the term is not just another name for physical or material stuff: "flesh is not matter, it is not spirit, it is not substance" [...] What is it? The *sensibility* of things, the perceptibility both of the perceptual environment and of ourselves as perceivers [...] That my body can be seen and touched is not just the empirical fact that I (or anyone) can be aware of it as an object; it is rather the underlying condition of my encountering and inhabiting a world at all in the first place [...] To see the world, we must already be in a kind of bodily communion with it.
>
> (Carman, 2020, pp. 115–116)

Having discussed, in the last chapter regarding Stein's concept of unfolding, the manner in which Gricoski stated he was using a relational ontology, explained as "a theory of being which places relationships at the ground level of metaphysics" (p. xviii), Merleau-Ponty's description of the embeddedness of our body in the world raises the image of relationship again for me, although he uses the idea of intertwining. Indeed, he links the ideas of flesh and chiasm in chapter four, 'The Intertwining – The Chiasm', in *VI.*

Carman suggests that although the concept of flesh is new in *VI* the concept of chiasm is not quite so new, because Merleau-Ponty's earlier interest in Gestalts was a precursor to, and similar to, the idea of intertwining in chiasm.

> A *chiasm* or chiasma is an x-shape or crisscross pattern; in grammar, a *chiasmus* is an inversion of parallel phrases, such as *When the going gets tough, the tough get going*, or *Working hard or hardly working?* And so it is,

> Merleau-Ponty believes, with body and world; they are not two distinct things, but sinews of a common flesh, thread in the same fabric, related to one another not as external situation and internal reaction, or stimulus and response, but as a single woven texture, like the interlocking birds and lizards in an Escher drawing.
>
> (Carman, 2020, p. 117)

As can be seen in this description, flesh and chiasm are interrelated since Merleau-Ponty suggests flesh is common to each of us and the world more generally. He says that the idea he is attempting to capture with the term "flesh" is not so much like "matter" but more like an element, "in the sense it was used to speak of water, air, earth, and fire, that is, in the sense of a *general thing*, midway between the spatio-temporal individual and the idea [...] The flesh is in this sense an 'element' of Being" (Merleau-Ponty, 1968, p. 139). However, the image of threads in the same single woven piece of fabric is one I find helpful when considering these concepts. I can imagine one thread within a piece of fabric being snagged or pulled and affecting the overall look and feel and experience of that piece of fabric. I can think of myself, and each of my service users, as a thread within a larger tapestry that is part of an even greater environmental tapestry. If one thread is hurt, the whole fabric is affected. This image is consistent with how Merleau-Ponty suggests each body engages in visual and tactile perception, as he provides examples of how our eyes move about and envelop what we perceive, and how as our left hand touches our right hand we experience both touching and being touched; to change the image, it is as if we are each part of a larger body as we are touched by, and touch, others. Any idea of rugged individualism and separate independent and purely cognitive experience does not stand up to his philosophical analysis. Indeed, the ease of the transmission of the COVID-19 virus and the ensuing global pandemic has also shone a light on the interconnectedness of us all on this planet.

These ideas of flesh and chiasm resonate with several ideas I presented in chapter three as I traced some of the changes in thinking about the soul over the last 2,500 years. The idea that we are embedded in the world, and share a common element with the world, is similar to Plato's descriptions of '"World soul" (*nous*)' and its connection with each individual's soul. Unlike Augustine's doctrine of 'original sin', Pelagius described 'original blessing', while Celtic spirituality more broadly considered a Divine spark in everything and the intertwining of the sacred in all of nature. Telehard de Chardin's form of spirituality considered humanity embedded in the material order and promoted a form of mysticism of involvement in the world, and William James' description of noesis involved a sense of oneness with all things. Thomas Moore more recently discussed the need for care of the World's soul, just as Ian Bradley has also suggested a recommitment to the Celts' ability to find God's glory throughout the natural world is necessary in order to save our environment from destruction.

Merleau-Ponty's phenomenology, relational ontology, and his examination of flesh within nature have led some philosophers to consider how these ideas might contribute to an ethic of care for the environment (Bannon, 2011). I appreciate how this project of reintroducing the language of the soul to narrative practices asks us to consider not only our own individual selves as a union of body-mind-soul, but also supports a call toward an ethic of care of others and the natural environment. This does not automatically occur since, as Bannon points out, considering that we and the rest of the natural order are intertwined and in relationship does not guarantee that people will then be drawn to care for nature and other people as they are more likely to have been caring for themselves, but rather might run the risk of them thinking they might as well take advantage of other people just as they have been stripping the world of its resources without consideration of the long-lasting effects. He says, "it is just as plausible, once human specialness has been questioned, to treat other humans in the instrumental manner in which natural beings are treated as it is to be more respectful toward a wider range of beings" (Bannon, 2011, p. 337). Bannon goes on to also explain that flesh should not be thought of as primarily the flesh of a human sensing body, and should not result in projecting onto, or anthropomorphizing, nature. He reiterates that the concept of flesh implies relations between bodies and that this flesh which is discovered between bodies actually holds them together (p. 345). He says,

> Merleau-Ponty calls the manner in which a particular body is open to its milieu a *dimension* and since consciousness is for Merleau-Ponty an embodied phenomenon, these dimensions can take on an intellectual or sensual character [...]: My body is an assemblage of relations that organizes its experience in a certain manner, according to the various dimensions through which it has access to a meaningful world. In the flesh of the human body, chiasmic relations fold over and create an interior dimension that we call consciousness, due to the way we behave given the specific relations between ourselves and other beings. While many other beings (e.g., mountains and rivers, not apes and lizards) do not exhibit these sorts of behaviours, we would be remiss to deny a kind of interiority to things: they still exist according to dimensions. However, to attribute interiority does not require the attribution of consciousness or even sentience.
>
> (Bannon, 2011, p. 347)

These ideas are similar to Stein's reflections on the body-soul union in all beings, and her point that despite this body-soul union, consciousness and a sense of 'I' does not necessarily occur in all beings. Nonetheless, Merleau-Ponty appears to be influenced by his interest in Gestalts, as Bannon explains Merleau-Ponty's work suggests "Gestalt is formed by the contact between field beings [... and] [a]s such a Gestalt, the flesh of the world reflects the distribution of beings within its field, but is not reducible to the sum of its parts" (2011, p. 349).

Bannon (2011) is particularly interested in examining what Merleau-Ponty's considerations can offer regarding a general environmental ethic. He contests arguments made by Abram, Toadvine, Barbara, and Dastur, who have interpreted Merleau-Ponty's ideas for an environmental ethic in a particular way, and then goes on to argue for the importance of not suggesting we return to a wild state of nature, nor that we anthropomorphize nature. Bannon suggests traditional forms of environmental ethics have focused on how far a moral concern should extend beyond human beings to non-human beings. He thinks it is more useful to move beyond an image of humanity and nature as being oppositional, taking up Merleau-Ponty's concept of flesh and chiasm, saying,

> Since human beings are inextricably part of the field of nature, the ethical debates should revolve less around how to preserve a nature without humans [a sort of wild pre-human nature] and more around how to engage with nature, how to leave a non-trivial space within nature for non-human forms of life, how to live with the changing face of the Earth's geology and atmosphere without attempting to master it, etc.
>
> (Bannon, 2011, p. 353)

Since we cannot help but affect those people, non-human beings, things, and the world in which we live, and since the effects we have on them will then have effects on us, it makes more sense to accept this and engage with one another with this awareness. Bannon goes on to suggest this means we can move away from having to choose between an ideal of removing traces of humanity from the world or accepting the human management of areas in which we attempt to preserve wilderness (not that this is a bad thing). Rather he says,

> We might even set as an aim the cultivation of wild places within our predominantly human places in order to re-welcome non-human forms of life and styles of living within our own communities and thereby enrich them. While there would no longer be any "pure nature," accepting the ecological vision of nature as flesh offers a different perspective upon the human presence within nature and richer possibilities for creating human lifestyles that are less speciesist and ecocidal.
>
> (Bannon, 2011, p. 354)

His related arguments regarding considering time and place differently (from an ecological versus purely human perspective) are compelling and remind me of some of my previous reflections on the Celtic spirituality's focus on the importance of place (Béres, 2012; 2013; 2017). Just as Teresa of Avila and Edith Stein's descriptions of human beings and their use of the language of the soul suggests turning inward and developing soulful contemplative practice should result in just actions in the world, so Maurice Merleau-Ponty's body phenomenology also extends far beyond a mere focus on the physical body or even the body-soul union. His deeply philosophical work has implications for psychotherapeutic work and socially just and ethical practices within our broader contexts.

Conclusion

Merleau-Ponty has said, "What Saint Augustine said of time – that it is perfectly familiar to each, but that none of us can explain it to the others – must be said of the world" (1968, p. 3). Time and perception are like 'taken-for-granted's that we do not often consider in our daily private and professional lives, but are part of how we engage with, and make sense of, the world. In exploring how we perceive the world, he describes looking at a table in the following manner:

> I must acknowledge that the table before me sustains a singular relation with my eyes and my body: I see it only if it is within their radius of action; above it there is the dark mass of my forehead, beneath it the more indecisive contour of my cheeks – both of these visible at the limit and capable of hiding the table, as if my vision of the world itself were formed from a certain point of the world. What is more, my movements and the movements of my eyes make the world vibrate – as one rocks a dolmen with one's finger without disturbing its fundamental solidity. With each flutter of my eye lashes a curtain lowers and rises, though I do not think for an instant of imputing this eclipse to the things themselves.
>
> (Merleau-Ponty, 1978, p. 7)

Having read this description, I cannot now forget this image of being able to be aware of my forehead, cheeks, and eyelashes as I look out at the world, nor how my eyes are constantly moving as they envelop the world. For me, these images and ideas reinforce the notion of my perception being due to my bodily place in the world. I've never accepted the idea of being able to be objective (with all that implies) but have realized my perspective is always subjective however much I attempt to bracket my presuppositions. Merleau-Ponty adds to this and reminds me that if this is true for me, this is also true for others in this shared fabric (or flesh) of this world. This requires, in therapeutic practices, spiritual direction, or pastoral counseling, a commitment to remembering the importance of the body-mind-world relationship; this relationship is consistent with, and possible to maintain while reintroducing, the language of the soul. My work with Eve, for example, as she became more comfortable with her trans identity and managed her anxiety in the world, would not have offered as respectful a therapeutic encounter if that encounter had not considered all layers and aspects of her whole 'true Self', or soul, including an awareness of the impact of her body on herself and her experiences in the world. Merleau-Ponty's image of chiasm, influenced by his interest in Gestalt psychology, offers a further image as we consider ourselves and the world as threads within a tapestry and each part affecting all the other parts. We are in relationship, in other words, and this notion of relationship and dialogue will be explored in detail in the next chapter.

Note

1 All names and identifying details of clients and case examples have been changed throughout this book.

References

Bannon, B. E. (2011). Flesh and nature: Understanding Merleau-Ponty's relational ontology. *Research in Phenomenology, 41*, 327–357.

Béres, L. (2012). A thin place: Narratives of space and place, Celtic spirituality and meaning. *Journal of Religion and Spirituality in Social Work: Social Thought, 31*(4), 394–413.

Béres, L. (2013). Celtic spirituality and postmodern geography: Narratives of engagement with Place. *Journal for the Study of Spirituality, 2*(2), 170–185.

Béres, L. (2017). Celtic Spirituality: Exploring the fascination across time and place. In B. Crisp (Ed.). *The Routledge Handbook of Religion, Spirituality, and Social Work* (pp. 100–107). Routledge.

Botelho, N. F. (2020). Reflection in motion: An embodied approach to reflection in practice. *Reflective Practice, 22*(2), 147–158.

Carman, T. (2020). *Merleau-Ponty, Second Edition*. Routledge.

Hersch, E. L. (2003). *From philosophy to psychiatry: A phenomenological model for psychology, psychiatry, and psychoanalysis*. University of Toronto Press.

Lefort, C. (1968). Editor's Foreword. In C. Lefort (Ed.) & A. Lingis (Trans.). *The visible and the invisible*. Northwestern University Press. (Original work published in 1964.)

Merleau-Ponty, M. (1968). In C. Lefort (Ed.) & A. Lingis (Trans.). *The visible and the invisible*. Northwestern University Press. (Original work published in 1964.)

Merleau-Ponty, M. (1978). C. Smith (Trans.). *Phenomenology of perception*. Routledge & Kegan Paul. (Original work published in 1962.)

Stein, E. (2002). K. F. Reinhardt (Trans.). *Finite and eternal being: An attempt at an ascent to the meaning of being*. ICS Publications. (Original work published in 1949.)

Stein, E. (2018). J. Koeppel, O.C.D. (Trans.). *The Science of the Cross*. ICS Publications. (Original work published in 1983.)

White, M. (2007). *Maps of narrative practice*. W.W. Norton.

Part III

Integrating the Language of the Soul into Postmodern Practice

7 I, Myself, and Bakhtin: Spiritual Direction and the Self

David Crawley

As described in the Introduction, my main areas of practice involve spiritual direction and pastoral care within Christian contexts, rather than therapy. Nonetheless, narrative ideas have continued to beguile me since I completed my narrative therapy training nearly 20 years ago. In this chapter, Laura has invited me to reflect on my experience as a spiritual director, including the ways in which the thought of Mikhail Bakhtin (1895–1975) informs my efforts to engage in 'soul work' from a narrative stance.

People who seek out spiritual direction, or other forms of spiritual care, such as chaplaincy or pastoral care, inevitably have stories to tell. Those engaged in spiritual care help them explore these stories in relation to their spiritual beliefs, uncertainties, and doubts. In approaching spiritual care from a narrative perspective, the greatest challenge for me has been the latter's discomfort with talk of the soul. In what follows, I will first describe my experience of this challenge in my own practice, before identifying some hopeful common ground between spiritual direction and narrative therapy. I will then describe how Bakhtin's dialogic literary theory has offered me a way to think and talk about matters of the soul without discarding narrative understandings of the fluidity and plurality of the self.

Spiritual Direction, Social Constructionism, and the Self

Within spiritual care conversations, when appropriate, I use familiar narrative practices such as externalizing a problem, mapping its effects, exploring what is absent but implicit, and listening for alternative stories of hope (White, 2007). Postmodern understandings of the role of social and discursive contexts in shaping identity and meaning have provided a helpful balance to intrapsychic models of personhood, which are strongly represented in the spiritual direction literature (Bidwell, 2009). Similarly, I have appreciated the freedom and creativity that accompany the non-essentialist understandings of the self which are embraced within narrative therapy.

The emphasis on the fluidity of the self, underpinned by social constructionist theory, has offered both freedom and challenge. There is

DOI: 10.4324/9781003137450-11

freedom from the never-ending quest to find an elusive true self. On the other side of that coin, however, is the challenge. For spiritual carers, it is commonly accepted that spiritual growth includes the development of a coherent, centered, core self. The tension between this assumption and social constructionist views of the self is articulated clearly by Ruffing (2012), an influential thinker and writer in the fields of Christian spirituality and spiritual direction. Having argued in earlier work (2011) for the helpfulness of approaching spiritual direction within a narrative frame, using Gadamer's hermeneutical theory, Ruffing critiques what she calls the "fragmented self" of postmodernism. Her own narrative paradigm allows for a degree of openness in the formation of the self: "An open story meets the future with flexibility, resilience in response to challenges and expects change and development over time" (2012, p. 66). Moreover, spiritual directors understand that God's activity may disrupt the coherent narrative of the self "by causing some kind of disorganization, contradicting an absolute form of self-assertion of the ego, or emerging as some inexplicable and mysterious confusion" (p. 70). Nonetheless, Ruffing's expectation is that spiritual directors will cultivate in themselves and those with whom they work "a coherent self that is capable of undergoing considerable transformation without becoming stranded either in fragmentation or rigid coherence" (p. 70).

As much as I find social constructionist accounts of meaning and identity philosophically compelling, *in practice* I find myself responding to people with language that embodies the notion of a coherent part of themselves, which some might call their 'core self' or 'soul'. I noticed this a few years ago when Susan[1] came for spiritual direction and spoke of her sense of confusion about a relationship which she had been in for some months. This uncertainty was making it difficult for her to concentrate at work and she was not sleeping well. She was unsure whether it was 'right' to continue the relationship, or not. 'I wonder', she mused, 'what God thinks of this, what God wants me to do?' My own silent wondering was less about what *God* wanted than what *Susan* herself really wanted here. Her sense of agency seemed thin. I suggested that it might be helpful to take some time to get away on her own, to reflect and pray: 'Perhaps it would be helpful to give yourself space to breathe, to put the worries aside for a while, to reconnect with your deeper self, and to consider whether or not this relationship is something that fits with the hopes you have for your life'.

As I reflected later on the suggestions I had offered to Susan, I noticed the alloy of narrative ways of speaking ('whether or not this relationship is something that fits with the hopes you have for your life') with notions of a 'deeper self' that holds important wisdom. I wondered how to reconcile these strands in my practice. Would it have been better simply to externalize confusion and explore its effects? To ask when Susan had been able to get the better of confusion, and what had enabled her to do that in the past? In hindsight, I think that this may have been helpful in supporting

Susan's agency, rather than inviting her to trust in my suggested approach. Eventually, however, I would still have come to a question that invited her to consider her own preferred path in this situation – to take a position, in narrative terms (White, 2007). At some point, she would need to consult that aspect of herself which holds her hopes and her vision for her life and decide. It was that aspect of herself which I had in mind when I referred to her 'deeper self'.

As I contemplate the relationship between my narrative training and my work as a spiritual director, two questions emerge. The first is whether narrative practices and spiritual direction share sufficient common ground to work together. Are there aspects of spiritual direction which are simply incompatible with the conceptual framework underpinning narrative therapy, as Ruffing suggests? The second question focuses more closely on the conceptual issue named in the reflections above. Is there an alternative theorization of the self that allows for both fluidity and a degree of coherence, a place for the language of the soul? The remainder of the chapter is woven around these two questions.

Spiritual Direction and Narrative Practices: In Search of Common Ground

Clarifying the Differences

The work of narrative therapy has been described as an *archaeology of hope* (Monk, Winslade, Crocket, & Epston, 1997), which is also an apt description of much of what takes place in spiritual direction. In recent years, therapists have become more aware of the importance of attending to their clients' spirituality, alongside other dimensions of their lives (Béres, 2017; Griffith & Griffith, 2003; Gubi, 2015). This has helped to narrow the gap between spiritual direction and therapy, yet differences remain. How spirituality itself is understood may be one point of difference. In chapter one, Laura observed that spirituality within therapeutic practice literature is often described as 'that which gives meaning and purpose to someone's life'. For those who seek out spiritual direction, spirituality generally also includes a transcendent element, an experience of something beyond the self, whether or not that something is thought of as divine (Swinton, 2010). Holloway and Moss argue that, within their own field of social work, spirituality needs to be an inclusive concept that "includes, but is not constricted by, religious world-views" (Holloway & Moss, 2010, p. 29). They therefore subsume religious understandings within a broader approach. Among those who come to spiritual direction, there are certainly some who identify as 'spiritual but not religious', but a greater number *do* hold beliefs of some kind. When it comes to people offering spiritual direction, most will also have their own religious beliefs, whatever their religion may be (Lommasson, 2005). Chaplaincy has historically operated from religious principles also, although more recently the case for secular and even atheist chaplains has been argued (Kolsen, 2017).

Understandings of spirituality aside, the most significant difference between spiritual direction and therapy concerns the focus and purpose of the work. On the one hand, while spirituality may increasingly be recognized as important in therapy, it is not the main focus. On the other hand, in spiritual direction, spirituality and spiritual experience will take center stage, sooner or later. Conversely, people do not come to spiritual direction primarily to talk about problems, although problems are often discussed. They come because of a desire to deepen their spirituality and to integrate it with the whole of their lives. For Ruffing, spiritual directors help others "with a personal understanding of the spiritual life, growth in self-knowledge, and deepening intimacy with God" (2011, p. 2). *Spiritual Directors International*, an inclusive, interfaith body, offers a broader description. The spiritual direction relationship is viewed as one which inspires people to experience authenticity in their lives "as they connect with and explore the ground of all being, that deepest of truths which is beyond life and death and goes by many names, including God, and no name at all" (Portrait of a spiritual director, 2018).

Unsurprisingly, soul language is ubiquitous in discussions of spiritual direction. A classic text in many spiritual direction training programs is entitled *Soul Friend: The Practice of Christian Spirituality* (Leech, 1980). More recent works on Christian spiritual direction include titles such as *Listening for the Soul: Pastoral Care and Spiritual Direction* (Stairs, 2001), *Spiritual Director, Spiritual Companion: Guide to Tending the Soul* (Edwards, 2001), and *Intensive Soul Care: Integrating Psychotherapy and Spiritual Direction* (Benner, 2005). In contrast, the language of the soul is virtually absent from the narrative therapy literature. This apparent reluctance to talk about the soul, the deeper self, the ground of being, or whatever language is preferred, is a challenge for those of us who want to apply narrative ideas to the work of spiritual direction, or spiritual care more generally. As observed in my reflections on working with Susan, I found myself calling on soul type language, even as I heard the voice of social constructionism in my head querying what I was doing! Thinking about this, I wondered whether narrative therapists sometimes find themselves drawing on similar terms. This sent me back to re-read some of Michael White's work, to see if he ever reaches for something approaching the language of the soul.

Spirituality and the Work of Michael White

Rather than engaging in conversations about a transcendent or ground-of-being kind of spirituality, White prefers, as Laura has pointed out in chapter one, to speak of "spiritualities of the surface" and "little sacraments of daily living". A careful reading of the context of White's use of these phrases suggests that he is thinking of times when people are reaching beyond "the accepted goals for life in this culture" (Hoyt, Combs, & White, 1996, p. 48). Spirituality, for White, seems to equate to "a knowing formation of the self according to certain ethics" (p. 36). He is careful to distinguish this understanding from spiritualities which reach for "an altitude above everyday life" or delve into psychological "caverns that are imagined deep below the surface of one's life" (p. 35).

A similar focus on ethical intention is evident when White elsewhere speaks of the importance of exploring what a person *accords value*, with a view to that value supporting them in the re-authoring of their identity. For example, in working with men who have perpetrated violence, he writes:

> We can proceed to trace the history of what the man accords value. These alternative values will fit with some other belief or idea about what it might be wise to do, and some other purpose or dream for life. These other values will not have come out of the blue, which is why historical inquiry is critical.
>
> (White & Denborough, 2011, p. 107)

In the same context, White writes about *resonance*, in relation to clients' experiences of trauma, and about the potential for experiences of resonance to reinvigorate a person's "stream of consciousness" or "language of inner life" (p. 123). Again, the focus here is on what is accorded value in a person's life, and what resonates with this in therapeutic conversation. Interestingly, White suggests that it is in these moments of resonance that a person recognizes their *self*, and it is this resonance "that contributes to the reinstatement of an 'I' in relation to 'myself'" (p. 127). He suggests that the exploration of a person's positive images of life and identity may set off reverberations with memories from the past, sponsoring "the development of an inner world that can be visualized, and a sense of aliveness that displaces a sense of emptiness and deadness" (p. 128).

Several things strike me about the language White uses here. First, terms such as 'dream for life', 'inner life', 'inner world', 'aliveness', 'resonance', and the sense of an 'I' in relation to 'myself', might easily have been excerpted from spiritual direction conversations. It is as though the challenges of working with people who have perpetrated violence, or experienced trauma, warrant the use of terms which White might otherwise prefer to avoid as being too close to depth metaphors. Second, what White seeks to address in the case of trauma is the fragmentation, loss or death of the person's sense of self. Certainly, he looks to history, memory, and story to account for the continuity and coherence of identity which a person may experience in the present, rather than the idea of recovering an essentialist true self. Nonetheless, I find echoes here of Ruffing's emphasis on supporting the development of a coherent self, and of the concern that found expression in my reference to a 'deeper self' in my spiritual direction conversation with Susan.

Finding Common Ground in Practice

These examples reinforce my sense that, however it might be named or imagined, the *practice* of narrative therapy does require reference to an aspect of the self, "an 'I' in relation to 'myself'", as White puts it, which is able to step back from the flow of lived experience to take a position in light of what is valued, and to make agentic decisions. In a review of narrative therapy's relationship to its espoused postmodern philosophical underpinnings, Polkinghorne argues that its focus on a creative and authorial subject renders it a hybrid of postmodern and existential ideas:

> The process of narrative therapy is built on the existential view that people have a capacity to revise and re-author the narratives in which they have been acculturated. The task of narrative therapists is to assist people in the exercise of this capacity [...] Narrative therapists believe in personal transformation through the generation of revised life stories. This belief separates these therapists from what has been the view of postmodern philosophers that the subject is a passive creation of social discourse.
>
> (Polkinghorne, 2004, p. 65)

If Polkinghorne's assessment of narrative therapy is accurate, then Ruffing's call to spiritual directors to practice in ways which support the development of a 'coherent self that is capable of undergoing considerable transformation without becoming stranded either in fragmentation or rigid coherence' is not substantially at odds with narrative therapeutic *practice*. Nor was my work with Susan significantly out of step with such practice, even if my structuralist language might not sit well with many narrative therapists.

On reflection, my reference to Susan's 'deeper self' was an in-the-moment metaphorical way of speaking of that aspect of her subjectivity which holds her hopes and intentions for life. It seems to me that White does something similar when he contrasts 'aliveness' in the 'inner world' with 'a sense of emptiness and deadness'. Presumably, this language also speaks to what is accorded value by White himself, in his work; namely, that which gives life. As an expression of this search for life, some narrative therapists embrace Deleuze's notion of "lines of flight" or "lines of life" in their work with clients (Duvall & Béres, 2011; Penwarden, 2018; Winslade, 2009). For Winslade, lines of flight are responses to the operations of power which are "directions rather than destinations and [...] lead to the living of life on some different plane or in some different territory" (2009, p. 338). He suggests that through Foucault's work on power, White found a therapeutic line of flight – a way to pursue the "spiritual struggle" (Winslade's description) for freedom from lines of power which "squeeze out the sense of being alive" (p. 338). This emphasis on moving toward freedom and life accords strongly with what spiritual directors and other spiritual carers hope for in their work with people. A key aspect of the work of spiritual direction is discernment. In accompanying another person on their journey through life, the director supports the other in discerning those paths, or stories, which most seem to lead *to life*.

I am not suggesting that White's language can be conflated with all that people engaged in spiritual conversations might mean by the soul. Some approaches to the soul reflect what White called 'immanent' forms of spirituality, which require delving within to find the true self. He explicitly distances himself from "a spirituality which is achieved by 'being truly and wholly who one really is,' 'by being in touch with one's true nature,' by being faithful to the god of the self" (Hoyt, Combs, & White, 1996, p. 35). Yet I find sufficient common ground here to feel hopeful about the project of integrating narrative therapeutic ideas with the work of spiritual direction.

Bakhtin's Dialogism and 'I' in Relation to 'Myself'

I turn now to my second main question. Are there non-essentialist ways of thinking about the self which allow for fluidity of identity and freedom from prescribed ways of being, while enabling practitioners to speak of something like a coherent inner life, which some might call the soul? In preceding chapters, Laura has responded to this question by drawing on insights from the contemplative tradition and Teresa of Avila – familiar territory for spiritual directors – as well as the history of philosophy and phenomenology, including Edith Stein's and Merleau-Ponty's ideas about the integral connection between body, soul, mind, and world. Others within the Christian tradition have approached the same question theologically (McFadyen, 1990; McMillan, 2017). In my own New Zealand context, some narrative practitioners are informed by Māori and Pacific understandings of personhood, within which spirituality is integral to life in all its dimensions: cultural, environmental, social, physical, and psychological (Crocket, Davis, Kotzé, Swann, & Swann, 2017; Mila, 2017; Waldegrave, Tamasese, Tuhaka, & Campbell, 2003).

Spending time with each of these approaches has enriched my appreciation of how narrative practice might acknowledge the importance of the inner life. When it comes to conceptualizing "an 'I' in relation to 'myself'", without resorting to essentialist notions of a true self, it is the dialogic literary theory of Russian philosopher Mikhail Bakhtin that has come to my aid. At the risk of over-simplifying his ideas, the rest of this chapter outlines aspects of Bakhtin's work which I have found helpful as I have wrestled with incorporating the insights and practices of narrative therapy with the work of being a 'soul friend' to others.

For Bakhtin, it is what takes place *between* people, whether in social or more immediate contexts, that shapes what takes place *within* persons. In his view, there are "no isolated acts in consciousness" (Clark & Holquist, 1984, p. 77). There are resonances here with Laura's account of Merleau-Ponty's work on perception: "it is as if we are each part of a larger body as we are touched by, and touch, others".

Bakhtin's Model of Subjectivity

How, then, does Bakhtin conceptualize human subjectivity? The answer is complex, but a good place to start is with his language of *I-for-myself, I-for-the-other,* and *other-for-me*. I-for-myself represents my sense of being a self which acts in the world. It is a fluid and diffuse locus of perception and identity. I-for-the-other names my sense of what the other sees of me, which is instrumental in forming my self-perception. Bakhtin insists that none of us can see or know ourselves without the involvement of the other. The other has an "excess of seeing" in relation to me and this is my only means of seeing myself (Bakhtin, Holquist, & Liapunov, 1990, p. 22). We are, Bakhtin suggests, "constantly and intently on the watch for reflections of our own life on the plane of other people's consciousness, and, moreover, not just reflections of particular moments of our life, but even reflections of the whole of it" (p. 16). Clark and Holquist offer a vivid description of what Bakhtin envisages here:

> The way in which I create myself is by means of a quest: I go out to the other in order to come back with a self. I 'live into' an other's consciousness; I see the world through that other's eyes [...] the mirror we use to see ourselves is not a passively reflecting looking glass but rather the actively refracting optic of other persons. In order to be me, I need the other.
>
> (Clark & Holquist, 1984, pp. 78–79)

Correspondingly, I have an excess of seeing in relation to the other, and my seeing of them helps to complete them. This is the *other-for-me*. This mutual shaping of subjectivity is at the heart of Bakhtin's dialogism. It gives rise to a dynamic, iterative understanding of identity formation. As Sullivan observes, "the various relationships of the self to others and itself are continually changing through their contact and interpenetration with each other" (2007, p. 109). There are echoes here of Merleau-Ponty's chiasmic metaphor, described in the last chapter, although the focus in Bakhtin remains primarily on what takes place between human beings, rather than extending to the non-human.

The fluidity and dynamism of this picture is consistent with social constructionist approaches to the self. Moreover, Bakhtin is aware that the voice of the other embodies a polyphony of voices, understood in terms of social discourse. Writing about the characters in Dostoevsky's novels, for example, he suggests that their every thought "senses itself to be from the beginning a *rejoinder* in an unfinalized dialogue [...] It lives a tense life on the border of someone else's thought, someone else's consciousness"

(Bakhtin & Emerson, 1984, p. 32). This polyphony calls to mind a social constructionist understanding of subjectivity as constructed within multiple discourses (Burr, 2015). Unlike most social constructionists, however, Bakhtin is interested in theorising the awareness which the self has of its own action. Sullivan suggests that this aspect of Bakhtin's work is sometimes missed:

> There is a tendency within current appropriations of Bakhtin's work to focus on one central hinge of his writings: how self and other shape each other through action. There is a second hinge or pole to dialogue, however, that tends to be overlooked. Bakhtin was also concerned with the sensation of self in action or how self looks and feels to its own consciousness in action.
>
> (Sullivan, 2007, p. 106)

It is in this aspect of Bakhtin's thought that I find a conceptual hook on which to hang White's reference to "an 'I' in relation to 'myself'". There is resonance here also with Laura's discussion of Stein's understanding of an 'I' that travels within a human being's layers, or within the inner mansions of the soul, as described by Teresa of Avila.

Spirit and Soul in Bakhtin

Intriguingly, Bakhtin sometimes employs the language of 'spirit' and 'soul' when differentiating aspects of the self. He was Russian Orthodox by background, but his use of these terms is metaphorical rather than religious and is intended to nuance his understanding of I-for-myself and I-for-other respectively. (This recalls the way Stein used 'spirit' and 'mind' interchangeably in describing the layers of human being.) I-for-myself, which Bakhtin sometimes refers to as spirit, is not an essentialist core. Rather, in terms of the earlier quotation, the spirit is that aspect of subjectivity which quests for meaning and self-knowledge; it goes "out to the other in order to come back with a self". It has no settled existence – it is not a fixed, true self – since "everything is yet-to-be for the spirit" (Bakhtin, Holquist, & Liapunov, 1990, p. 110).

In contrast to the open, questing nature of the spirit, soul, for Bakhtin, is "the aesthetically valid whole of a human being's inner life" (Bakhtin, Holquist, & Liapunov, 1990, p. 132). This is the sense of self which is dependent on "another's loving activity from outside its own bounds" – the I-for-other (p. 132). As psychotherapists Griffith and Griffith (2003) suggest, we can gain a one-dimensional view of ourselves from a mirror, but "what we need is an aesthetic interpretation"; the question, "How do I look?" is "a hint of our need to know how we are experienced in the consciousness of another" (pp. 109–110). Through the words, actions, and emotional responses of the other, the potentiality of the spirit is given form and value, and this is what Bakhtin refers to as soul.

In chapter five, Laura drew attention to Stein's suggestion that human beings begin their lives lacking the capacity for self-reflection, until the I/spirit is awakened to understanding and choice. Bakhtin has a similar developmental understanding when it comes to the I-for-myself:

> The words of a loving human being are the first and most authoritative words about him; they are the words that for the first time determine his personality *from outside*, the words that *come to meet* his indistinct inner sensation of himself, giving it a form and name in which, for the first time, he finds himself and becomes aware of himself as a *something* [...] and it is in her love that his first movement, his first posture in the world is formed.
>
> (Bakhtin, Holquist, & Liapunov, 1990, p. 50)

The words 'in her love' highlight the dialogic nature of the process – it is in the mother's love that the child begins in its own turn to act upon the world. Similarly, in adult life, the way I address myself to another and the world is already informed by their excess of seeing of, and actions toward, me. The I-for-myself, therefore, is both formed *by* the other (I-for-other) and gives form *to* the other (other-for-me). As Holquist suggests, we "must share our mutual excess in order to overcome our mutual lack" (in Bakhtin, Holquist, & Liapunov, 1990, p. xxvi). In this way, human beings are continually engaged in the mutual co-authoring of identity.

Alongside this picture of the dialogic formation of subjectivity, I want to introduce some further Bakhtinian ideas which I have found particularly congenial to narrative practice and its application to soul work.

Dialogization, Authoritative Discourse, and Internal Persuasion

Bakhtin's understanding of language is integral to his dialogic understanding of personhood: "Where there is no word and no language, there can be no dialogic relations" (Bakhtin, Holquist, & Emerson, 1986, p. 117). Every word which enters our external or internal conversations carries with it a history of others' usage and meanings. Like identity, therefore, language and meaning are dialogic. Bakhtin argues that

> there are no 'neutral' words and forms – words and forms that can belong to 'no one'; language has been taken over, shot through with intentions and accents. [...] The word in language is half someone else's. It becomes 'one's own' only when the speaker populates it with his own intention, his own accent, when he appropriates the word, adapting it to his own semantic and expressive intention.
>
> (Bakhtin & Holquist, 1981, p. 293)

Just as there is no purely self-made person – we are formed in and through dialogic encounter – so there is no word or utterance which does not invisibly reference a host of earlier utterances by other speakers. When participants in a conversation use a word like 'God' or 'spirituality' (or 'soul'!) in common, they bring to the interaction their own meanings, each laden with its own history. For Bakhtin, "a word, discourse, language or culture undergoes 'dialogization' when it becomes relativized, de-privileged, aware of competing definitions for the same things" (Bakhtin & Holquist, 1981, p. 427). Encountering another's meaning has the potential to *dialogize* my own, adding richness and new layers of significance, and inviting me to reconsider taken for granted understandings. Narrative practitioners will recognize this as an aspect of the deconstruction of dominant discourses, which in therapeutic contexts is intended to help clients recognize their personal agency and the possibility of choice (Béres, 2014, p. 49).

The opposite of dialogization, for Bakhtin, is *authoritative discourse*; that is, speech which attaches one meaning to a word, as if there were no contending interpretations (1981, p. 427). When this happens, an interaction or conversation becomes *monologic*, rather than dialogic. Then, according to Bakhtin, "the genuine interaction of consciousnesses is impossible" (Bakhtin & Emerson, 1984, p. 81). Authoritative discourse, he argues, "is by its very nature incapable of being double-voiced [...] there is no space around it to play in" (Bakhtin & Holquist, 1981, p. 344). In the therapeutic context, Anderson suggests that

> Dialogical space refers to room in one's thoughts to entertain multiple ideas, beliefs, and opinions. [...] Dialogical space or conversational context is critical to the development of a generative process that promotes fluid, shifting ideas and actions. [...] Without dialogical space a familiar story cannot be narrated in a way that provides an opportunity for transformation in the narrating story and the self.
>
> (Anderson, 1997, pp. 112–113)

This suggests that truly dialogic engagements will be marked by creativity, spontaneity, and the freedom to play with narratives that have claimed authoritative status.

Monologic encounter can assume subtle forms. A conversation may have the appearance of dialogue, but if one party sets the terms and offers the interpretation of what is said, then the process is monologic rather than dialogic. I have written elsewhere about how spiritual direction conversations can subtly take on a monologic character (Crawley, 2016). I am indebted to my narrative training for sensitizing me to the ways in which therapists and other helping professionals are often positioned with considerable power by the discourses of our social contexts. In religious settings, a further layer of power is added when clergy and carers are regarded as having a divine mandate, or insider access to divine guidance. Even the term spiritual director is somewhat power-laden, harking back to an era when it applied to the superiors of monastic communities. Despite the disclaimers we make about this terminology to those we work with, spiritual directors are susceptible to invitations to speak on God's behalf – as when Susan wondered aloud, "I wonder what God thinks of this, what God wants me to do?" In enticing moments like these, I try to maintain White's (2005) de-centered and influential posture, to ensure that the conversation remains dialogic rather than monologic. Bakhtin's understanding of dialogism in terms of the mutual authoring of our souls is a reminder that genuine encounter is never neutral. I therefore appreciate the term "influential" as a reminder to ensure that primary authorship status remains with the other (White, 2005, p. 9).

Another aspect of Bakhtin's thought provides some reassurance for practitioners concerned about their own influence: Whether an encounter is monologic or dialogic, the developing I-for-myself does not automatically assimilate the other's meanings, or excess of seeing. As noted earlier, a child's development beyond dependence on a parent's authoritative input is marked by an increased agency and capacity for dialogic engagement with the meanings offered by others. Those meanings which people *do* assimilate as their own are described by Bakhtin as *internally persuasive*. The I-for-myself capacity for discrimination develops as people encounter difference and engage in an internal dialogue with what is offered to them. I find another suggestive connection here with Laura's exposition of Stein's phenomenology, when she notes the latter's argument that 'there is a certain type of understanding that can strike more deeply than the intellect, engaging the whole human being/the whole soul'.

Bakhtin's theorization of the self therefore makes room for both a measure of coherence, associated with internal persuasion and the formation of the soul, and a fluid openness toward the future, reflected in the always yet-to-be of the spirit. This leads to another of Bakhtin's key ideas: the unfinalizability of the self.

Unfinalizability and Agency

Even where internal persuasion occurs, the assimilated meaning is not fixed, but subject to new and creative variations. Bakhtin argues that the "semantic structure of an internally persuasive discourse is *not finite*, it is *open*; in each of the new contexts that dialogize it, this discourse is able to reveal even newer *ways to mean*" (Bakhtin & Holquist, 1981, p. 346, [italics in original]). This statement evokes for me Geertz's phrase, "it is the copying that originates", cited by White and Epston (1990, p. 13) in relation to "the indeterminacy of texts" and the creative possibilities inherent in re-authoring conversations.

As indicated already, the I-for-myself, or spirit, resists finalization. As Bakhtin (Bakhtin, Holquist, & Liapunov, 1990, p. 127) observes, "I cannot count and add up all of myself, saying: this is *all* of me". The fullness of who I am is not yet seen; it is always yet-to-be. It follows that, while we are dependent on others for our sense of self, we can at the same time recognize that neither they nor we have spoken the last word concerning our lives or identities. This *unfinalizability* of the self, as Sullivan points out, is a source of hope:

> The author of action is always felt as being more than just the action, so he or she also exists in the future as a felt potential. Hence, while, as beings with 'soul', we may feel responsible for an action (i.e., injuring someone), we also, as beings with 'spirit', feel the potential of redemption in the future.
>
> (Sullivan, 2007, p. 112)

In chapter one, Laura drew attention to Guilfoyle's acknowledgment that human beings overflow their "discursive imprisonment". In connection with this idea, Guilfoyle (2015, p. 119) explicitly refers to Bakhtin's account of unfinalizability, noting the negative effects on others of finalizing forms of relationship. I had the opportunity to hear stories of such effects – physical, emotional, psychological, and spiritual – in the course of doctoral research interviews with people who had experienced sustained monologic practices of religious authority. I think of Selina, for example, who recalled describing her embodied experience of these practices to a friend in this way: "I said to her, 'I feel like I've been presented with this very, very, very shallow coffin that I'm being asked to lie down in. And I don't think I can fit my body in there'" (Crawley, 2014, p. 143). The participants also told stories of eventually resisting these practices and their finalizing tendencies. In Deleuzian terms, their narratives traced lines of flight toward life. In language inspired by Bakhtin and Stein, this might also be viewed as an uprising of the spirit – the unfinalizable I-for-myself, which, in Stein's words cited by Laura in chapter five, "cannot be captured in static definitions, but must rather be a continual movement seeking fluid expression" (Stein, 2018, p. 112).

In my life and my practice, Bakhtin's notion of unfinalizability challenges me to consider the way in which the other lives in my imagination. There are many ways in which finalizing attitudes can creep into spiritual direction practice. Popular psychological theories (including personality profiles) may be used to categorize people. I may slip into limiting assumptions about the other, concerning their ethnicity, gender, sexual orientation, or physical abilities. It requires effort to relate to each person's story and spiritual experience as unique and unfinalizable. Writing of the stance required of spiritual directors, Guenther observes that "The person sitting opposite me is always a mystery. When I label, I limit" (1992, p. 19).

As Sullivan and McCarthy note, unfinalizability "gives us a certain agency in the social world or in changing our self-interpretations" (Sullivan

& McCarthy, 2004). While a child unconditionally accepts the sense of identity formed through her mother's words and action, these remain authoritative. But, as she grows in awareness of other voices and actions, her mother's responses will be weighed against those of others and the sense that she is something more, something yet-to-be, will grow. Holquist observes that the I-for-myself acts "as the seat of perception and ground for action" (in Bakhtin, Holquist, & Liapunov, 1990, p. xix). In therapeutic terms, we might recognize this as the seat of agency. It is, in terms of the narrative metaphor, the authoring self, which, although it is dependent on the co-authoring responses of others (I-for-other), is not completely defined by those responses. I recognize here an aspect of subjectivity for which I was reaching in referring Susan back to her 'deeper self'. In her anxiety about making the "right" choice, I felt that she had a thin sense of her own agency/author-ity in her decision making (Crawley, 2016). The depth metaphor is problematic for some, and I wonder how better to language this 'I' in relation to 'myself', which sifts meanings and exercises agency on behalf of a yet-to-be consummated vision for life. It might be called the heart, the soul, the spirit, or the inner self. In the end, it is the client's preferred way of languaging this aspect of themselves, rather than mine, which matters. If, like Laura's client Eve (in chapter six), someone I am working with finds it helpful to speak of their 'true Self', my inclination to dialogize this language needs to take a back seat!

Answerability and Bakhtin's Ethic of Love

While there is reassurance for practitioners in Bakhtin's notions of internal persuasion and unfinalizability, the influence we have as co-authors still carries an ethical responsibility, and this too is an important element in Bakhtin's work. His account of the dialogic process by which identity and meaning are co-authored is not a dispassionate analysis, but a statement of ethical responsibility. As Sullivan observes, for Bakhtin, "perceiving or authoring the other is an ethically charged *act* that is emotionally responsive to the needs of the other" (2007, p. 110).

Answerability is a term used by Bakhtin in connection with this ethical responsibility. I answer the other, out of my excess of seeing, and at the same time I am answerable *to* the other – open to their response, to knowing myself as their other-for-me. *How* we engage in this process of mutual formation is critical for Bakhtin. In a word, his is an ethic of *love.* Specifically, this means actively paying lovingly interested attention to the other: "The valued manifoldness of Being as human [...] can present itself only to a loving contemplation" (Bakhtin, Liapunov, & Holquist, 1993, p. 64). This is incompatible with any finalizing gaze which views the other "in light of a prefabricated category" (Jacobs, 2001, p. 30). It is also at odds with passivity and indifference. Bakhtin observes that a response to another's speech which "remains purely passive, purely receptive contributes nothing new to the word under consideration, only mirroring it [...] in no way enriches the word" (Bakhtin & Holquist, 1981, p. 281). In terms of answerability, such a response is an ethical failure because it leaves the original speaker "in his own personal context, within his own boundaries" (p. 281). There is a twofold loss in such passivity, since it also deprives the listener of the possibility of receiving a reciprocal response from the speaker (Jacobs, 2001, p. 37).

Bakhtin's ethic of lovingly interested attention challenges any tendency I have as a practitioner to play it safe by offering only reflections and summaries in response to the other's story. Such responses are an important part of listening well, and I am grateful for my early training in these skills. Yet I recall my narrative therapy tutor challenging me to go beyond this non-directive approach – to be influential in the re-authoring process, while remaining de-centered. White advocates an approach which "engages people with others in ongoing revisions of their images about who they might be, and about how they might live their lives" (White in Hoyt, Combs, & White, 1996, p. 37). He is clear that, because of the impossibility of neutrality, practitioners are right to distrust what they are "for" in terms of imposing their own ways of life and thought (p. 39). Positively, however, as they engage in "double-listening" (an aspect of Bakhtin's excess of seeing), they can help people notice and address what is sabotaging their lives. They can encourage people

> to attend to some events of their lives that just might be of a sparkling nature – events that just might happen to contradict those plots of their lives that they find so unrewarding and dead-ended [...] to join with people in the exploration of the knowledges and practices of life that might be associated with these alternative plots.
>
> (Hoyt, Combs, & White, 1996, p. 39)

I never had the opportunity to meet Michael White in person, but in watching videos of his work with people I observe him doing just this. I find myself wondering how he sees or hears things in their stories which he perceives to be of a 'sparkling nature'. The excess of seeing out of which he responds is no finalizing diagnosis. He is careful to check out with the client(s) whether what he notices is something that they are for, rather than assuming this. Sometimes he opens a line of enquiry which proves not to be internally persuasive for the client(s), in which case it usually fades from the conversation. This requires humility on our part as practitioners, and a willingness to hold our noticing lightly. Interestingly, during the conversation from which these quotations are drawn, the interviewer says to White, "I was very moved by the eloquence of your presentation this afternoon. I thought it was *practical love*. That's what came to mind: *love in practice*" (Hoyt, Combs, & White, 1996, p. 34, [italics in original]). With some qualifications, White agrees. He suggests that "we need to be reclaiming these sorts of terms in the interpretation of what we are doing – *love, passion, compassion, reverence, respect, commitment*, and so on" (p. 34, [italics in original]).

As indicated earlier, part of my dissatisfaction with looking to social constructionism alone as a theoretical basis for narrative practice related to its conceptualization of the self. Additionally, I have found social constructionism to be a thin basis for ethical practice, although it can certainly be used as a powerful tool toward an ethical end. In chapter 2, Laura reflects on what it means in life and practice to hold together an experience of "complex fluid identities as well as an ongoing coherent and ethical sense of the self". Bakhtin's notion of loving answerability, integral to his dialogic understanding of meaning and identity, helps me to live that dialectic in a way that I find both philosophically satisfying and ethically challenging.

Bakhtin and the Divine Other

As someone who identifies with the Christian tradition, I find it interesting to consider what formed Bakhtin in his ethic of attentive love. Felch and Contino (2001) find its source in his Russian Orthodox background. Jacobs suggests that, for Bakhtin, it is the Incarnation of Christ, the divine Word become flesh, that "provides the ground for, or source of, my own determination to act answerably" (2001, pp. 39–40). By his own account, Bakhtin (Bakhtin, Holquist, & Liapunov, 1990) finds in Christ "an infinitely deepened *I-for-myself* [...] one of boundless kindness toward the other" (p. 56). Through Christ, God is revealed to be no longer simply "the voice of my conscience", but the one who is loving, merciful, and accepting of me. "What I must be for the other", writes Bakhtin, "God is for me" (p. 56). As a child's first posture in the world is formed in its mother's love, so the ethic of loving acceptance ultimately has its ground in the "boundless kindness" of the divine Other. This is answerability in its highest form:

> Only un-self-interested love on the principle of 'I love him not because he is good, but he is good because I love him,' only lovingly interested attention, is capable of generating a sufficiently intent power to encompass and retain the concrete manifoldness of Being, without impoverishing and schematizing it.
>
> (Bakhtin, Liapunov, & Holquist, 1993, p. 64)

It follows that the un-self-interested love I receive from the other is key to knowing myself in ways that are not impoverished or schematized. The quest of the I-for-myself to know itself as an 'aesthetically valid whole' may therefore be profoundly realized in the I-for-*Other*, where this Other embodies a divine quality of love and seeing. Griffith and Griffith point this out, with Bakhtin's ideas in mind:

> Only God can witness all of me as a person [...] One can think of "God" as an epistemological position to which a person moves when it is important to witness the whole of one's life. This self-reflective knowing often takes place through prayer and during meditation [...] If people are conversing with or being counselled by an Other who fully knows them, knows the hearts of people around them, and knows their past and future, then it might enrich our conversation to give ear to this Other.
> (Griffith & Griffith, 2003, pp. 109–110)

Not all clients – not even all of those who come for spiritual direction – believe in God in any conventional religious sense. Griffith and Griffith suggest that people may nonetheless have their own ways of moving to this "epistemological position" (2003, pp. 110–112). They tell the story of a client for whom it was the spirits of her deceased grandparents who knew her, comforted her, and offered her wisdom. Narrative therapists will recognize parallels here with the practice of engaging clients in re-membering conversations (Hedtke & Winslade, 2004; White, 1997).

The kind of self-reflective knowing described here by the Griffiths names something of what I hoped for when I suggested to Susan that she might find it helpful to step back from her impasse, to reconnect with her 'deeper self'. Because I had sensed in her story a picture of a God who would weigh her decision, and a fear that she would be found wanting, I steered away from God-language in my suggestion. Yet, as Bakhtin argues, there is no deeper self which is completely independent of the other/Other. The soul with which we may commune in quiet moments is gifted to us and formed through countless dialogic encounters. Some of these formative encounters are loving and helpful, while some are negative and sabotaging of our quest for life. For me, recalling the place of the world and the body in Merleau-Ponty, positive formative encounters have often involved the natural world, as well as other people, texts, music, art, and a transcendent sense of the Divine. My hope for Susan was that in prayerful solitude there might be opportunity to sift through the polyphony of voices informing her I-for-other awareness and to connect with those which resonated most with the vision she held for her life (I-for-myself), whether or not she recognized in these the voice of her God. I am struck by the similarity here with White's idea of spirituality as a "knowing formation of the self according to certain ethics", cited earlier.

In hindsight, I think it may have been helpful first to talk more about what 'God' meant for Susan. Bakhtin's dialogic understanding of language is a reminder of the multiple meanings which attach themselves to such words. In such a conversation, we might have explored some of those meanings for Susan. From my own excess of seeing, I might have wondered aloud with Susan what effects some of these meanings were having on her ability to make a decision based on love rather than fear. Taking up the idea of God as an epistemological position to which one can move when it is important to have a sense of one's life as a whole, I might then have explored with Susan how best to connect with that quality of self-knowledge – with her soul.

Conclusion

Laura's intention in this book has been to explore the language of the soul, with a view to contributing to 'ongoing and fluid' discussions about human existence and addressing a perceived gap in the theorization of narrative therapy. In this chapter, I have reflected on the common ground which I experience between spiritual direction and narrative therapy, as well as naming an area of tension around the conceptualization of the self and the language of the soul. I have presented some ideas from Bakhtin's dialogic literary theory which have offered me language to speak about the self/soul/spirit, in ways that feel congruent with my formation in both spiritual direction and narrative therapy. As Laura has emphasized, this book is not primarily about ontology or structure – the soul as a *thing* or *place* within a person – but about language. Indeed, part of the gift of Bakhtin's dialogism and his call to an ethic of love (answerability) is to direct our attention to what happens *between*, rather than simply *within* persons.

By holding together I-for-myself, I-for-other, and other-for-me, Bakhtin offers language for what is implicit in narrative practice, namely the idea that each person holds values and a vision for their life in the world, and that others in their life have an integral place in the formation and thickening of these hopes and values. This conceptualization enables me to converse with another of what it might mean to care for, nourish or listen to their own soul, without collapsing the latter with an essentialist, autonomous or fixed self. This might mean seeking a quiet space in which a polyphony of voices can be sifted, spending time in nature (Lydia in chapter one), reading poetry or Scripture, listening to music, talking with a friend, reconnecting with one's culture/ancestors, cultivating silence and stillness, engaging in contemplation, or any number of other practices.

Finally, for those whose spirituality includes a sense of the Divine, connecting with that aspect of our being which we might call the soul may sometimes lead to encounter with a mystery that transcends even our implicit knowing. On rare occasions, when my own well of hopes and dreams has run dry, I have been gifted with an internally persuasive word, originating, as it has seemed to me, from a Divine Other's excess of seeing: "You are loved"; "Don't be afraid"; "I am with you"; or, as to the medieval mystic Julian of Norwich (2015, p. 75), "All will be well".

Note

1 All names and identifying details of clients and case examples have been changed throughout this book.

References

Anderson, H. (1997). *Conversation, language, and possibilities: A postmodern approach to therapy*. BasicBooks.

Bakhtin, M. M., & Emerson, C. (1984). *Problems of Dostoevsky's poetics*. University of Minnesota Press.

Bakhtin, M. M., & Holquist, M. (1981). *The dialogic imagination: Four essays*. University of Texas Press.

Bakhtin, M. M., Holquist, M., & Emerson, C. (1986). *Speech genres and other late essays* (V. McGee, Trans.). University of Texas Press.

Bakhtin, M. M., Holquist, M., & Liapunov, V. (1990). *Art and answerability: Early philosophical essays* (V. Liapunov, Trans.). University of Texas Press.

Bakhtin, M. M., Liapunov, V., & Holquist, M. (1993). *Toward a philosophy of the act* (V. Liapunov, Trans.). University of Texas Press.

Benner, D. G. (2005). Intensive soul care: Integrating psychotherapy and spiritual direction. In L. Sperry & E. P. Shafranske (Eds). *Spiritually oriented psychotherapy* (pp. 287–306). American Psychological Association.

Béres, L. (2014). *The narrative practitioner*. Palgrave Macmillan.

Béres, L. (Ed.). (2017). *Practising spirituality: Reflections on meaning-making in personal and professional contexts*. Palgrave Macmillan.

Bidwell, D. R. (2009). The embedded psychology of contemporary spiritual direction. *Journal of Spirituality in Mental Health, 11*(3), 148–171. 10.1080/19349630903080947

Burr, V. (2015). *Social constructionism* (3rd ed.). Routledge.

Clark, K., & Holquist, M. (1984). *Mikhail Bakhtin*. Harvard University Press.

Crawley, D. R. (2014). *Stories of resistance to religious authority: A discursive analysis*. [Doctoral thesis, The University of Waikato]. The University of Waikato Research Commons. https://hdl.handle.net/10289/8665

Crawley, D. R. (2016). Authority in spiritual direction conversations: Dialogic perspectives. *Journal for the Study of Spirituality, 6*(1), 6–19. 10.1080/20440243.2016.1158452

Crocket, K., Davis, E., Kotzé, E., Swann, B., & Swann, H. (Eds). (2017). *Moemoeā: Māori counselling journeys*. Dunmore Publishing.

Duvall, J., & Béres, L. (2011). *Innovations in narrative therapy: Connecting practice, training, and research*. W.W. Norton.

Edwards, T. (2001). *Spiritual director, spiritual companion: Guide to tending the soul*. Paulist Press.

Felch, S. M., & Contino, P. J. (2001). *Bakhtin and religion: A feeling for faith*. Northwestern University Press.

Griffith, J. L., & Griffith, M. E. (2003). *Encountering the sacred in psychotherapy: How to talk with people about their spiritual lives*. Guilford Press.

Gubi, P. M. (Ed.). (2015). *Spiritual accompaniment and counselling: Journeying with psyche and soul*. Jessica Kingsley Publishers.

Guenther, M. (1992). *Holy listening: The art of spiritual direction*. Cowley.

Guilfoyle, M. (2015). Listening in narrative therapy: Double listening and empathic positioning. *South African Journal of Psychology, 45*(1), 36–49. 10.1177/0081246314556711

Hedtke, L., & Winslade, J. (2004). *Re-membering lives: Conversations with the dying and the bereaved*. Baywood Publishing Company.

Holloway, M., & Moss, B. (2010). *Spirituality and social work*. Palgrave Macmillan.

Hoyt, M. F., Combs, G., & White, M. (1996). On ethics and the spiritualities of the surface: A conversation with Michael White. In M. F. Hoyt (Ed.). *Constructive therapies* (Vol. 2, pp. 33–59). Guilford Press.

Jacobs, A. (2001). Bakhtin and the Hermeneutics of Love. In S. M. Felch & P. J. Contino (Eds). *Bakhtin and religion: A feeling for faith* (pp. 25–45). Northwestern University Press.

Julian of Norwich. (2015). *Revelations of Divine Love* (B. A. Windeatt, Trans.). Oxford University Press.

Kolsen, M. (2017). Atheist hospital Chaplains: The time has come. *American Atheist, 55*(2), 19–21.

Leech, K. (1980). *Soul friend: The practice of Christian spirituality.* Harper & Row.

Lommasson, S. (2005). Widening the tent: Spiritual practice across the traditions. In S. M. Buckley (Ed.). *Sacred is the call: Formation and transformation in spiritual direction programs.* Crossroad.

McFadyen, A. I. (1990). *The call to personhood: A Christian theory of the individual in social relationships.* Cambridge University Press.

McMillan, L. (2017). Social God, relational selves. In L. McMillan, S. Penwarden, & S. Hunt (Eds). *Stories of Therapy, Stories of Faith* (pp. 3–17). Wipf & Stock Publishers.

Mila, K. (2017). Mana Moana: Healing the *Vā*, developing spiritually and culturally embedded practices. In L. Béres (Ed.). *Practising spirituality: Reflections on meaning-making in personal and professional contexts* (pp. 61–78). Palgrave Macmillan.

Monk, G., Winslade, J., Crocket, K., & Epston, D. (Eds). (1997). *Narrative therapy in practice: The archaeology of hope.* Jossey-Bass.

Penwarden, S. (2018). *Conversations about absence and presence: Re-membering a loved partner in poetic form.* [Doctoral thesis, The University of Waikato]. The University of Waikato Research Commons. https://hdl.handle.net/10289/12102

Polkinghorne, D. E. (2004). Narrative therapy and postmodernism. In L. E. Angus & J. McLeod (Eds). *The handbook of narrative and psychotherapy: Practice, theory, and research* (pp. 53–68). Sage.

Portrait of a spiritual director. (2018). *Presence: An International Journal of Spiritual Direction, 24*(4), 40–41.

Ruffing, J. K. (2011). *To tell the sacred tale: Spiritual direction and narrative.* Paulist Press.

Ruffing, J. K. (2012). Spiritual identity and narrative: Fragmentation, coherence, and transformation. *Spiritus, 12*(1), 63–74. 10.1353/scs.2012.0016

Stairs, J. (2001). *Listening for the soul: Pastoral care and spiritual direction.* Fortress Press.

Stein, E. (2018). *The Science of the Cross.* (J. Koeppel, O.C.D., Trans.) ICS Publications. (Original work published in 1983.)

Sullivan, P. (2007). Examining the self-other dialogue through 'spirit' and 'soul'. *Culture & Psychology, 13*(1), 105–128. 10.1177/1354067x07073662

Sullivan, P., & McCarthy, J. (2004). Toward a dialogical perspective on agency. *Journal for the Theory of Social Behaviour, 34*(3), 291–309. 10.1111/j.0021-8308.2004.00249.x

Swinton, J. (2010). The meanings of spirituality: A multi-perspective approach to 'the spiritual'. In W. MacSherry & L. Ross (Eds). *Spiritual assessment in healthcare practice* (pp. 17–35). M & K Publishing.

Waldegrave, C., Tamasese, K., Tuhaka, F., & Campbell, W. (2003). *Just therapy – a journey: A collection of papers from the Just Therapy Team, New Zealand.* Dulwich Centre Publications.

White, M. (1997). *Narratives of therapists' lives.* Dulwich Centre Publications.

White, M. (2005). *Workshop notes*. Retrieved 16 April 2020 from www.dulwichcentre.com.au

White, M. (2007). *Maps of narrative practice*. W.W. Norton & Co.

White, M., & Denborough, D. (2011). *Narrative practice: Continuing the conversations*. W. W. Norton & Co.

White, M., & Epston, D. (1990). *Narrative means to therapeutic ends*. Norton.

Winslade, J. (2009). Tracing lines of flight: Implications of the work of Gilles Deleuze for narrative practice. *Family Process*, *48*(3), 332–346. 10.1111/j.1545-5300.2009.01286.x

8 Possibilities Offered: Weaving the Language of the Soul into Narrative Practices

Laura Béres

Had I the heavens' embroidered cloths,
Enwrought with golden and silver light,
The blue and the dim and the dark cloths
Of night and light and the half-light,
I would spread the cloths under your feet:
But I, being poor, have only my dreams;
I have spread my dreams under your feet;
Tread softly because you tread on my dreams.[1]
W.B. Yeats (1865–1939)

For several years I have been suggesting the need to carefully incorporate the area of spirituality into professional helping practices, and in this book I have been presenting the language of the soul as providing a possible way to fill what I have experienced as a 'gap' in the postmodern and social constructionist therapeutic modality of narrative therapy. However, I can at times make this project fraught with anxiety for myself, not only due to how dear it is to me, but also due to knowing how important the underlying philosophical and political values of narrative therapy are to practitioners, which might make some hesitant to consider the ideas I have presented regarding the soul and spirituality. Ideas from two quite different books have influenced how I have chosen to move ahead as I weave together concepts reviewed in previous chapters: The first book, *Narrative in Social Work Practice: The Power and Possibility of Story* (2017), is a collection of essays written by social workers with training in both narrative therapy (White & Epston, 1990) and narrative medicine (Charon, 2006); The second book, *Reimagining the Sacred* (2016), offers a series of dialogues about Richard Kearney's concept of 'anatheism'. I will begin this chapter by discussing the ideas presented in these two books since they provide a way forward, imagining what a dialogue about the language of the soul and narrative practices might entail, particularly focusing on ideas from *Reimagining the Sacred*. I will highlight some of the material from previous chapters, suggesting how the language of the soul may contribute to the theoretical foundations of narrative therapy and a respect for the

DOI: 10.4324/9781003137450-12

complexity of 'finite human being'. I will also present some thoughts about adding the time and space for silence and contemplation within narrative practices, concluding with how these ideas link to the potential for 'human flourishing' (Gaye, 2010). Maintaining an openness to dialogue about these philosophical ideas must involve a willingness to engage with uncertainty and an ongoing deconstruction of notions like 'center' or 'depth' of the self. With my wishes for this project in mind, I have included Yeats' poem as an epigraph for this chapter; a colleague and former supervisor, Denis Costello, framed a copy of this poem for his therapy office, explaining that he would gesture to it when meeting with people for the first time, suggesting he thought of what they shared in his office as their dreams, and that he would commit to 'tread softly'. The ideas I am bringing into dialogue are important to many people (Christian, spiritual but not religious, and secular practitioners) and I also wish to tread carefully.

As I immersed myself in the works of Teresa of Avila, Edith Stein, and Merleau-Ponty and wrote about their conceptions of the soul I have often thought, and made comment, of how consistent some of their ideas are with some of the postmodern and social constructionist ideas within narrative therapy: there are overlaps, as in a Venn diagram. However, this is despite the fact there has been little language of spirituality and no language of the soul in narrative therapy's theoretical base until now, and despite the fact some narrative therapists may remain hesitant about considering making a place for the language of the soul within their practice. Nonetheless, I believe Michael White, as one of the originators of narrative therapy, would have been interested and supportive of how I imagine the inclusion of the language of the soul within narrative practices. At the conclusion of his training workshops and conferences, I often heard him encourage participants to try some of their new narrative practice skills without fear of needing to 'get it right', or 'be just like him'. As David mentions in the last chapter, White and Epston have previously quoted Geertz and his idea of "copying that originates" (Geertz in White & Epston, 1990, p. 13), and this is what White would remind us of in workshops. He reassured us that even imitating always also involves an element of creation and that he would have been interested in learning how our narrative practices evolved over time. Certainly, through bringing Teresa of Avila and Edith Stein as well as Maurice Merleau-Ponty and Mikhail Bakhtin into a dialogue with narrative therapy, these practices cannot help but evolve.

One of the aspects of *Narrative in Social Work: The Power and Possibility of Story* (2017) that intrigues me is the manner in which, despite seemingly different philosophical positions (the medical field based on scientific research with the stance of doctor as expert, alongside a postmodern therapy with a decentered but influential stance), practitioners from both narrative medicine and narrative therapy have been able to learn from one another and dialogue about their practices. An editor and contributor, Burack-Weiss, comments in her acknowledgments that one of the rewards of a long career as a social worker is "[s]eeing the pendulum of theory and practice swing back and forth – each time bringing part of the past along with it, each time moving the needle a bit forward" (Burack-Weiss in Burack-Weiss, Lawrence, & Bamat Mijangos, 2017, p. XVII). Certainly, by adding the language of the soul to narrative therapy, the pendulum will continue to move. In her introductory chapter, Burack-Weiss goes on to explain how the narrative perspective, through White and Epson's narrative therapy, had a great influence in social work, particularly in relation to questioning the 'therapist as expert', and demonstrating how mental health professionals could assist people in authoring their own preferred storylines "that focus on strengths and potentials rather than on deficits and limitations" (Burack-Weiss in Burack-Weiss, Lawrence, & Bamat Mijangos, 2017, p. 8). She then acknowledges the work of Rita Charon, the founder of the program in Narrative Medicine at Columbia University, who provides concrete methods for professionals to maintain and develop skills in empathic engagement with others' stories: Close reading and reflective writing being the two primary methods used in this approach. Both fields took a narrative and creative turn, but in different contexts and with different backgrounds, but nonetheless were able to learn from one another. The collection of chapters provides an honoring of White and Epson's work as well as Charon's, showing how each can be enriched by the other. In the Foreword, Charon comments that the chapters hold in common "the fierce joy of helping a person to recognize the meaning of the tale he or she tells, the narrative humility of opening to the *mystery of the other* [italics added], the reflected trauma of witnessing the suffering of others, and the soft echoes of self and other within the immersive listener" (Charon in Burack-Weiss, Lawrence, & Bamat Mijangos, 2017, p. IX). I will come back particularly to this theme of 'mystery of the other'.[2]

In *Reimagining the Sacred* (2016), Richard Kearney first provides a summary of his concept 'anatheism' and then, in the following chapters, engages in a series of dialogues about this concept with various theologians and philosophers, from Charles Taylor (Roman Catholic philosopher), Catherine Keller (feminist and eco-theologian), and David Tracey (Roman Catholic theologian), on the one hand, to Julia Kristeva, and Simon Critchley, (both atheist philosophers), on the other. Kearney's description of anatheism, as well as the presentation of dialogue between theists, atheists, and secular humanists, provides a useful structure also for considering the process of how to speak of the soul in the primarily 'post-Christian', 'after-God', context of a postmodern therapeutic practice like narrative therapy.

Anatheism as an Aid to Dialogue

Kearney (who could be described as a postmodern Christian philosopher) begins his summary of anatheism by presenting the Shorter Oxford English

Dictionary definition of the prefix 'ana': "Up in space or time; back again, anew" (Kearney, 2016, p. 6). He goes on,

> Thus, in the prefix *ana-* we find the idea of retrieving, revisiting, reiterating, repeating. But repeating *forward*, not *backward*. It is not about regressing nostalgically to some prelapsarian past. It is a question, rather, of coming back "afterwards" in order to move forward again [...]. So, it is in this sense that I use the term *anatheism* as a "returning to God after God" [during our current time that is often described as more secular]: a critical hermeneutic retrieval of sacred things that have passed but still bear a radical reminder, an unrealized potentiality or promise to be more fully realized in the future.
>
> (Kearney, 2016, p. 7)

For Kearney, it is important that 'ana-theism' contains both 'theism' and 'atheism'. From whichever position a person begins, as either theist or atheist, the suggestion is that they let go of, or bracket, their beliefs and then re-engage with ideas about God – and I would add ideas about spirituality, and the language of the soul – without any judgment about which is the better position in which to end. He suggests that he, and other anatheists, may continue to shift between more theist beliefs at some times, and more atheist beliefs at others. I find this concept of anatheism, and the process of engaging with these big questions in life, refreshing and helpful in relation to considering concepts of the soul. As Tyler (2016) has shown, and as I have presented in chapter three, the language of the soul has always been complex, and has been taken up with a different focus in different times and contexts. In hoping to reintroduce the language of the soul into postmodern therapeutic practice this description of anatheism provides an image of how it might be possible to go back to examine what is an ancient idea of the soul, and, more specifically, Teresa's writing about the soul in the 1500s, and then Stein's, Merleau-Ponty's, and Bakhtin's further developments regarding ways of considering the body-soul-world relationship, including perception and experience, during the 1900s, while also bringing them forward in time and examining them with fresh eyes for what they can contribute to postmodern (or even post-postmodern, as Finlay, 2009 suggests) narrative practices. As Kearney says, anatheism "operates from a space and time *before* the dichotomy of atheism and theism, as well as *after*. The double 'a' of *anatheism* holds out the promise but not the necessity of a second affirmation once the 'death of God' has done its work" (Kearney, 2016, p. 7). This sounds like a postmodern perspective as it unsettles the either/or approach to people's thinking about the Divine. Kearny says, "[a]natheism concentrates, therefore, on unrealized or suspended possibilities, which are more powerfully reanimated if one also experiences a moment of a-theism – the 'a-' here being a gesture of abstention, privation, withdrawal" (p. 8). He calls upon the language of the 'dark night of the soul' which Stein reflects upon in *The Science of the Cross* (2018), which I discussed in chapter five; this process of letting go of, or bracketing, ideas and beliefs can feel like stepping into a void or a liminal space, as I suggested, and yet is always followed by something else and the possibility of a fresh new dawn. This does not mean, as I have stated above, that Kearney is only looking at a path of spiritual maturing that is 'meant' to result in theism. Anatheism, rather, provides a way of making space for dialogue between people of varying faiths and nonfaiths, since it supports movement away from any form of dogmatism. Since narrative therapy was developed as a postmodern secular approach to counseling and I am bringing two Christian mystics (as well as Merleau-Ponty and Bakhtin) into dialogue with narrative therapy's theorists, the dialogical process offered by anatheism will be helpful. This asks us to phenomenologically bracket any ideas of soul we might have, and then reconsider them. Some of us might take up the language of the soul again or for the first time, and some might not, but merely considering it can be a useful process, aiding in dialogue, and enriching whichever position we choose to take. This will also assist us in developing a comfort with, and competence in, working with these ideas should people in counseling contexts be interested in them.

Despite our secular age, people continue to search for the sacred and the spiritual, if not the religious. In recognizing this, Kearney also suggests that 'anatheism' is an attempt to sacralize the secular and secularize the sacred. It is reimaging the sacred after the secular and through the secular. Bonhoeffer [(1906–1945), a Lutheran pastor and theologian], talks about being *with* God yet living *without* God" (Kearney, 2016, p. 17). This always involves unpacking any ideas we develop about God, or the soul, any time they become fixed or dogmatic. Kearney suggests a fixed idea becomes like a fetish that needs to be deconstructed, whereas he suggests considering these as more fluid ideas and holding on to them tentatively. He summarizes this in the following manner:

> [T]he anatheist God is one of perpetual departing and arriving, conjoining negative capability with constant rebirthing of the divine in the ordinary. For me, this double sense of leaving and returning is at the heart of the sacred. And it may express itself either spiritually (as a general gracious openness to "something more") or religiously (involving creedal commitments and devotions). Anatheism has many mansions. One can be either an anatheist theist or an anatheist atheist, but whichever one chooses – belief or nonbelief – anatheism remains a wager.
>
> (Kearney, 2016, p. 17)

As I have said elsewhere (Béres, 2017) and in earlier chapters, introducing spirituality and the language of the soul to therapeutic practices should not involve proselytizing nor dogmatism. Therapeutic practitioners should also retain an open nondogmatic stance willing to engage with areas of life and belief that are important to those people consulting them, and that will at times mean ensuring space for spirituality and the language of the soul.

Kearny and Critchley, in their chapter, "What's God? 'A Shout in the Street'", suggest "Critchley's atheist transcendence aligns with Kearney's anatheism on [the] level of faith as a wager rather than a certainty" (Kearney & Zimmerman, 2016, p. 150). Having been asked whether he is saying that religious writers can tell us 'more' about humans than non-religious writers, Critchley answers that is what he is saying if the non-religious are liberal humanists "wedded to an idea of progress based on a faith in scientific development – for me that is a 'theological' dogma that needs to be confronted and challenged by something like faith" (Critchley in Kearney & Zimmerman, 2016, p. 152). He goes on, "it's a question of trying to recover the subtlety, complexity and depth of thinking about the human that one finds in genuine religious thinkers" (p. 152). As I've quoted Charon stating above, narrative therapy and narrative medicine, although not influenced by any religious faith, open us to the "mystery of the other" (Charon in Burack-Weiss, Lawrence, & Bamat Mijangos, 2017, p. IX). Narrative therapists, as postmodern practitioners, also problematize the certainty and dogma that are part of modern scientific rationality, and so, perhaps, are positioned well to listen to the mystics who have explored the complexity of human being and transcendence. As David has indicated in chapter seven as he described Bakhtin's work on dialogue, narrative practitioners' therapeutic posture and commitment to the two-way process of therapeutic engagement offers the type of dialogue that supports the authorship, knowledge, and beliefs of the person consulting us and which is required for conversations about spirituality and the soul.

In another chapter, Kearney and Keller engage in a dialogue entitled "Beyond the Impossible". Catherine Keller is described as a professor of constructive theology, "a process theologian with wide-ranging theoretical interests, encompassing feminist theology, ecotheology, and post-structuralist and postcolonial theory" (Kearney & Zimmerman, 2016, p. 46). Her work combines theology and science, drawing on quantum physics to move beyond modernist views to consider interconnectedness within the universe, which resonates with Merleau-Ponty's focus on flesh and chiasm and the manner in which these ideas have been taken up in consideration of the environment. She states:

> I see anatheism as operating on three main axes, each a kind of chiasmic interchange. First and most obviously, it oscillates between theism and atheism; second, it forms a crossover between Christianity and non-Christianity (which includes [...] not just Judaism and Islam but also, vividly, Buddhism and Hinduism); and thirdly, there is a chiasmus between apophatic interiority and kataphatic outreach into action – outward ethical and political praxis.
>
> (Keller in Kearney & Zimmerman, 2016, p. 47)

These three axes she presents are consistent with themes I have raised in earlier chapters of this book and can easily be woven into a narrative therapist's stance and practice. There is space within narrative practices for a wide range of faiths, theisms, and atheism. Narrative practice is also committed to dialogic rather than monologic conversations and is committed to socially just practices. However, perhaps there is room to incorporate more contemplative, or "apophatic interiority" (Keller in Kearney & Zimmerman, 2016, p. 47) into narrative practices, and I will return to this idea later in this chapter.

The Narrative Therapeutic Posture and the Importance of Dialogue

Building upon the above arguments regarding the need for dialogue, White (1997) has critiqued what he describes as the traditional one-way account of therapy, which supports the image of a service user 'in need' meeting with a therapist who possesses expert knowledge that can be provided in a one-way flow. He suggests, alternatively, that a two-way account of therapy will "transgress the oft-made work/life boundary distinction" (p. 132) – not in an unethical manner, overstepping professional boundaries – but, rather, in such a way that acknowledges that we cannot bear witness to other peoples' efforts and not be affected emotionally and intellectually by them. David, in the last chapter and in Crawley (2016), has discussed similar ideas when he draws upon Bakhtin's literary theory, describing further nuances in the distinctions between monologue and dialogue. David explains that "at the heart of Bakhtin's theorization of language and texts is an emphasis on the dialogic (double-voiced) character of all language and language use" (Crawley, 2016, p. 8). Bakhtin, therefore, suggests all meaning-making is necessarily dialogic, but then meanings 'jockey for position' and one person's meaning may be seen to have more authority than another's. As David has also distinguished in the last chapter, in this way language can be dialogized or used in an authoritative manner: "a word, discourse, language or culture undergoes 'dialogization' when it becomes [...] de-privileged, aware of competing definitions for the same things" (Bakhtin and Holquist in Crawley, 2016, p. 9). As David has explained, a spiritual director, for example, may want to discuss 'God' in a dialogized manner, acknowledging how the word contains multiple meanings, and Tyler (2016) has certainly shown the various ways in which 'soul' is used as a signifier.

I believe White's acknowledgment of the two-way process of engaging with people in conversation, and Crawley's reminder of the dialogic manner in which words and language operate, create a space for postmodern therapeutic practitioners to participate in a dialogue about the language of the soul. As Critchley points out, this type of conversation requires that everyone involved takes a nondogmatic stance and is willing to examine ideas which might previously have been discarded. I am hopeful that this is possible. This acknowledgment of the shifting nature of meaning within language also resonates well with Tyler's (2016) comment that "soul language is the language of the choreography of the transcendent and the immanent" allowing for a way of seeing the physical and spiritual at the same time, so that neither is overemphasized (p. 181). I appreciate this choreography image, since this suggests an acceptance of the movement within language, and within the specific word 'soul', while also gesturing toward the embodiment of the soul.

Spirituality of the Surface, Little Sacraments of Daily Existence, and the Embodied Soul

In chapter one, I described White's interest in the "spirituality of the surface", or the "little sacraments of daily existence" (2000, p. 145), although he otherwise did not have a professed practising spirituality or religious faith. David also drew upon these same interests of White's in the last chapter. In chapter one, I further presented Guilfoyle's arguments regarding the importance of considering ourselves "embodied" and "in flow" (2014, p. 132). Although these ideas could be read by some as privileging the material over the spiritual soul, they do not need to be. Tyler's (2016) work, as well as the work of both Teresa of Avila and Edith Stein, indicate that the language of the soul can include the physical, while Merleau-Ponty's work particularly focuses on the embodied soul. Teresa and Stein do not privilege the soul over the body, and their work suggests that the soul and body are in fact one entity, with the soul perhaps animating the body but both body and soul developing and changing overtime and affected by social interactions. In fact, Stein, using the image of the Trinity, suggests the body, soul, and spirit are three-in-one. Teresa and Stein both also argue, despite a commitment to their internal spiritual lives, that practices like Quiet Prayer (contemplative, or apophatic, prayer as described in chapter two) are only truly worthwhile if socially just acts flow from them into the world: As Teresa argues, referencing the biblical story of Mary sitting at Jesus' feet, while Martha toiled in the kitchen, there needs to be a balance of both Mary-like and Martha-like behaviors in our lives. We need time to 'unplug', 'recharge', or just contemplate, as well as then act in the world from a reflective position grounded in our personal values.

In order to ground some of these reflections in a practice example, I will briefly describe my work with Vicky.[3] Vicky is a middle-aged cis-gender woman and single mother who experienced several losses in her childhood, followed by ten years in a heterosexual marriage characterized by control, manipulation, and degradation. She told me she had received counseling in the past that focused on her experiences of intimate partner violence and the process of leaving the matrimonial home safely and accessing therapeutic supports for her child. She said that she now wants to focus on herself in counseling appointments with me, wanting to experience some hope and happiness again in her life. She commented at one point in her second session with me that her issues and concerns have been so great that she has not found that focusing on her breathing to be very helpful, as had been suggested to her by previous counselors, she said. I totally agree with her. Despite the interest and research regarding incorporating mindfulness into various therapeutic modalities, merely suggesting someone focus on their breath without any context as to why this might be useful could seem minimizing of their concerns. I also believe that narrative therapy's curiosity regarding people's meaning-making, values, and preferences is often a crucial first step before any incorporation of discussion of practices related to spirituality, mindfulness, or 'apophatic interiority', unless they raise these practices themselves.

Indeed, one of the strengths of narrative therapy's theory and practice is that therapeutic conversations remain focused on assisting people in examining their meaning-making and articulating their personal values and preferences for living – rather than diagnosing, prescribing, or even rushing to problem solving or offering of suggestions, like the suggestion to practice breath-work. Assisting people in examining and evaluating the effects in their lives of their interactions in the world, which have been influenced by those meaning-making activities and values, can then result in people being able to make their preferred changes in life, while some people will want to discuss matters of a more spiritual nature. Although I have found the therapeutic posture of narrative therapy, the privileging of curiosity over certainty, and the focus on supporting people in re-authoring their lives, can be useful when people raise spiritual issues, my narrative practices have been further enriched by Teresa's and Stein's conceptions of the soul, alongside reminders from Merleau-Ponty and Bakhtin regarding the importance of remembering the soul is embodied, entwined within the environment in relationship and in dialogue. Using the image of layers of the human being (Stein, 2000) or mansions of the soul (Teresa of Avila, 2013), remembering these are merely images or metaphors, rather than normalized structures against which to judge a person's insights, will be particularly helpful for these narratively informed therapeutic conversations about spirituality and the soul. Vicky suggested she had needed to first of all focus on issues related to her context, environment, and areas which could be described as outer layers, or outer mansions, but now has been raising a wish to pursue areas more related to her inner layers or inner mansions.

Layers of the Soul/Human Being

Teresa provides a beautifully poetic description of her experiences of 'layers of herself' as she describes her soul as an 'interior castle' with many mansions. Her descriptions are those of a mystic attempting to capture some of her experiences in otherwise limiting everyday language. Narrative therapists, perhaps borrowing skills in close textual reading from narrative medicine, might be able to engage with her writing with empathy and curiosity regarding the soul and perhaps transcendent experience also. Her descriptions of the various mansions within the interior castle, with each providing different experiences, are similar to Stein's ideas of layers of human being. Stein's work certainly built on Teresa's ideas of outer mansions of the soul being more influenced by the physical and social world (and the social construction of identity), and inner mansions offering the possibility to gradually provide distance from the distractions of the world and finally the experience of mindfulness, contemplation, and possibility of a relationship with the Divine. As described in chapter five, Stein, in her earlier work, *Philosophy of Psychology and the Humanities (PPH)* (2000), suggests there are phenomenal realms related to four different layers of a human being: the physical, the sentient, the mental, and the personal. Her descriptions of these layers show that she was already moving beyond any dualism of body and soul, placing these realms all within the body, "where all four express what is ordinarily termed the soul as well" (Sawicki, 2000, p. XV).

In chapter one, I explained that White and Epston (1990) suggest the "positivist physical sciences", "biological sciences", and various approaches within "social sciences" all use varying metaphors which then have an impact on how problems and solutions are constructed. Rather than using machines or organisms, which would then focus on attempting to find the cause of a problem and then have an 'expert' attempt to correct it, they were more interested in the analogy of text and the possibility of people re-authoring events to move into the performance of preferred storylines. However, in addition to this, I pointed out that White also said at a later stage that he had perhaps overly emphasized the power of constructed stories over our lives, because he also did not believe people "go about life [...] mindlessly re-enacting or reproducing these stories [...]. Stories provide the frames that make it possible for us to interpret our experience, and these acts of interpretation are achievements that we take an active part in" (White, 1995, p. 15). As I also pointed out, he does not, however, discuss how it is possible for there to be a part of a person that has agency and the ability to actively resist a particular story, discourse, or socially constructed sense of self. Stein's and Merleau-Ponty's conception and description of 'I' provides one possible way of considering how this might be possible.

Stein's (2000; 2002) description of the experience of the 'I' (or consciousness) moving about within the various layers of human being is useful when considering how an element of the self can be active and aware of other aspects of the self. She says, once the 'I' has been awakened in a human being, the 'I' is able to examine events and respond to them "in personal freedom [...] People do not, however, make full use of their freedom but rather abandon themselves to a large extent – much in the manner of merely sentient creatures – to the pressures and forces of external and internal 'events' and 'drives'" (Stein, 2002, p. 370). She goes on, drawing directly from Teresa's work, saying that the soul "as an interior castle, is like a space with many mansions in which the I is able to move freely, now going outward beyond itself, now withdrawing into its own inwardness" (Stein, 2002, p. 373). I suggest much of the literature about narrative therapy has until now been primarily focused on describing the practice of working with people who want to change aspects of their lives that could be considered as being influenced by the outer layers of the self, which is obviously of utmost importance and often related to their safety, as in Vicky's earlier experiences of counseling. However, narrative practitioners are also able to engage in therapeutic conversations about inner layers of the self if they are willing to be open to conceptualizations of the complexity and mystery of human life beyond the use of the metaphor of text and the social construction of identity.

As I explained in chapter five, Stein suggests that the 'I' can begin to study the soul as an object even though the 'I' and the soul are closely related. She goes on to say that the soul takes part in a call and response process (such as dialogue and consistent with Bakhtin's work), resulting in a person choosing to act in a certain way, to make a stand, or to take a position based on the meaning made of a particular context (Stein, 2002, p. 439). To narrative therapists, these activities will all sound consistent with their practices – particularly the process of inviting people to take a position in relation to externalized problems and initiatives. Stein, however, also goes on to say,

> The personal I is most truly at home in the innermost being of the soul. [...] In this interiority the I is also closest to the meaning of every event, most open to the demands with which it is confronted, and in the best possible position to evaluate the significance and the import of these demands. Few human beings, however, live such 'collected' lives. The [I] of most of them takes a stand on the surface.
>
> (Stein, 2002, p. 439)

Although some might read this as judgmental, and as suggesting that people 'should' live more 'collected' lives, narrative practitioners can allow these ideas to assist them in joining with people in conversations about their own preferences for their spiritual journeys, rather than imposing some ways as more highly valued than others. In Stein's conceptions, the soul works to develop itself and form the material body, but it also has the opportunity, through an ever-deepening or inner journey, to become more than that through a relationship with the Divine, but this is always done within the context of free will. For Stein, as for Teresa, this inner journey involves a movement toward something like a 'center'.

Without calling upon this idea of 'center', and in being curious about what was sustaining her, I asked Vicky if she was engaged in any form of spirituality. She said she had been taken to church as a child but had lost all hope in life through her early losses. She said that she felt that she was born into life to suffer and then die. I could certainly hear her despair and felt 'invited', or drawn, to also experience that despair, but I could also hear Michael White in the back of my mind talking about the 'absent but implicit' and how when people complain about an absence of hope this means they have had some experience of hope in the past and are taking a stand against ongoing hopelessness. I, therefore, became interested in Vicky's past experiences of hope and present glimmers of potential hope and peace through an exploration of unique outcomes – previously unstoried events in her life. She was able to describe moments when she sits in her garden looking at the trees or shuts out intrusive thoughts by listening to music. These activities appear to help her 'be in the moment' and settle herself more effectively than any direction to slow or follow her breath has in the past. Her activities that kept her in the moment were linked to her own skills, knowledge, and experience rather than suggested by an external expert.

Continuing to Unsettle the Language of Depth and 'Center'

Returning to the notion of 'center', narrative practitioners do not use the language and metaphors of depth nor center in relation to people, since they argue these are related to particular discourses that privilege Western notions of individuality as well as implications that there is some 'true' inner self to be found. Without a close reading of the works of mystics such as Teresa of Avila and Edith Stein, the work of body phenomenologist Merleau-Ponty and literary theorist Bakhtin, as well as the work of academics like Tyler (2016), non-religious and non-spiritual therapists are likely to expect the language of the soul to come with dogmatic beliefs and directions as to what is 'right'. This need not be the case and even when Teresa and Stein describe their experiences and conceptions of the inner mansions of the soul, and the idea of a 'center', they are describing these in a fluid, unstructured manner. As Tyler (2013) points out, for Teresa, the center is there and not there, as she radically deconstructs any preconceived notion of the self. Williams (1991) also argues that Teresa's approach does not keep people wedded to a notion of individual self, but rather has them moving beyond it. Merleau-Ponty expands these possibilities further, truly arguing for the weaving of the 'I' into the whole of creation through his concepts of 'flesh' and 'chiasma'. With these ideas in mind, I can imagine how it is so many people like Vicky experience this connection with nature as something spiritual. If as Teresa, Stein, and Merleau-Ponty suggest, we can conceive of the various aspects of ourselves, like 'I', body, and 'soul', interwoven and layered and then also interwoven with the rest of the cosmos, there are certainly multiple ways of engaging with someone in therapeutic and spiritual direction conversations.

Adding Silence and Contemplation to Narrative Practices

As an academic, with an interest in philosophical and spiritual literature, it is probably understandable that I am drawn to theory, knowledge creation, and hence people's meaning-making behavior. Prior to receiving any training in narrative therapy, when I was a young clinical social worker beginning my career, a supervisor pointed out that she thought I had natural abilities in engaging people in cognitive restructuring: an important aspect of cognitive behavioral therapy (CBT). Although I am familiar with CBT, and may at times incorporate elements of it into my primarily narrative therapy practice, I do not consider myself a practitioner of CBT. However, looking back, I think I may have at times overly privileged cognitive elements within my narrative practices, as I demonstrated a curiosity in how people made sense/meaning of their experiences. I have been fascinated in assisting people in deconstructing internalized discourses, and I took to heart Michael White's concerns that emotions no longer be privileged or prioritized in therapeutic settings. His suggestion that we ask someone what is in their teardrop if they could unpack it, rather than merely asking them how they were feeling as they cried, has led to wonderfully rich conversations about both emotions *and* their cognitive reflections on what contributed to those emotions.

I have primarily worked with adults in therapeutic contexts, and so my experiences have offered numerous opportunities for conversations rich with meaning-making and cognitive/rational explorations. However, my experience and focus are not the only experience possible within narrative therapy and certainly not a necessary focus of narrative practices. For instance, many narrative practitioners work primarily with children and engage in much more creative and playful manners in their therapeutic work (e.g., Freeman, Epston, & Lobovits, 1997). In a similar vein to my slippage into using a cognitive focus in narrative work at times, as I began to explore ways in which to integrate spirituality into therapeutic practices, and began to argue for the need to expand bio-psycho-social assessments into bio-psycho-social-spiritual assessments, I also inadvertently over emphasized aspects of definitions of spirituality which highlighted the manner in which it provides a sense of meaning and purpose in people's lives. Again the 'meaning' element seemed to overemphasize a cognitive ability to make a judgment about what is meaningful in a person's life. This may have been due in part to presenting these ideas within a university context where I was teaching social work students, and where it often feels safer to stress the cognitive and rational. However, there is much more to the spiritual and the therapeutic than the cognitive, and emotional. One recent experience of being involved in a research project regarding what attracted people with dementia to a therapeutic gardening program highlighted the need for me to ensure space for more than just rational exploration.

A very popular therapeutic gardening program is offered in a local setting that offers day care programming for people with a diagnosis of dementia who otherwise continue to live at home with their carers in the community. Shortly after the expansion of the gardening area and the subsequent development of the therapeutic gardening program, Hall, Mitchell, Webber, and

Johnson (2018) examined the effects of the gardening program on well-being among participants. Following the completion of what was a mixed methods study which highlighted positive effects of therapeutic gardening, and due to the program continuing to generate interest from participants with dementia, a colleague and I were invited to assist the developer of the program in exploring what it was about therapeutic gardening that participants enjoy. We wanted to hear from participants themselves to gain a greater understanding of how they might describe their experiences and the ways in which gardening in this context contributes to their well-being. We employed an Interpretative Phenomenological Analysis (IPA) approach to this study since it is particularly well-suited for exploring how individuals make sense of their lived experiences, providing deep and rich descriptions of their *meaning-making*. Several themes emerged from the data, ranging from "Activating the sense of touch", through "Reminiscence of past gardening" to "Social benefits". Two additional themes that emerged, "Finding meaning: Curiosity, wonder, and lifelong learning" and "'It's just another season': Cultivating peace and hope" contained elements related to spiritual effects for participants (Smith-Carrier, Béres, Johnson, Blake, & Howard, 2019). Interestingly, our experiences as a multidisciplinary research team required us to move beyond initial expectations of our chosen IPA methodology and to include studies of spirituality in order to enrich our analysis of the data. It became clear, for instance, that although focusing on the meaning-making element contained within definitions of spirituality might make the term more palatable for non-spiritual and non-religious service providers, only focusing on what could be perceived as a cognitive skill of meaning-making would have severely limited our understanding of the data. Indeed, Daly, Fahey-McCarthy, and Timmins (2019) demonstrate through their systematic review of the literature that people living with dementia, who are experiencing cognitive challenges, continue to experience the "ongoing importance of spirituality [...] as a means of finding hope, meaning and linkage with past, present and future" (p. 448). Indeed, spiritual experiences can encompass all aspects of a person, and we were interested to see that gardening was one way in which a person could engage with a sense of spirituality. Some of the participants indicated this was due to making connections to happy memories of working in gardens in the past, noticing the passing cycles of the growing year, and making links to their own cycles of life, or just being in the moment as they focused on the what the plants needed, based on the weather conditions and state of the earth. Supporting people's connection to their gardens, and to nature more broadly (even Vicky's love of sitting in her back garden looking at the trees) engages with other layers of themselves which are not always acknowledged in talk therapy. Another area that can seem almost at odds with the whole notion of 'talk' is that of silence, and yet it can be useful to consider ways in which to incorporate silence into narrative practices.

Although mindfulness practices have already been incorporated into practices like dialectical behavior therapy (DBT), mindfulness-based-cognitive therapy (MBCT), and acceptance and commitment therapy, Blanton (2007) suggests the benefits of considering also adding contemplation to narrative therapy, while also pointing out the following:

> Stories refer to what people tell about themselves, and stories present clients' understanding of the meaning of their life events. Stories depend upon language. On the other hand, silence alludes to the process of disengaging from both internal and external dialogue. In silence, one quiets the language-processing areas of the left hemisphere of the brain.
>
> (Blanton, 2007, p. 212)

He goes on by quoting Siegel and asking, "Why silence?", and explaining that silence provides the stillness and space to become intimate with one's mind, and I would suggest soul. "When we start a journey to attune to our own minds by pausing into stillness we enter a realm of experience that can produce surprise in each moment" (Siegel in Blanton, 2007, p. 212). He asks how contemplative practices might enlarge narrative therapy.

Much as I have done in earlier chapters, Blanton first points out that people who contemplate are often referred to as mystics, going on to explain that mystics often experience "everything as a unified whole", losing a sense of a separate individual identity, experiencing time differently, as well as feeling awe, love, peace, and joy (Blanton, 2007, p. 213). He goes on to also draw upon William James' *The Varieties of Religious Experience* (1902) and points out that mystics' experiences are often difficult to put into words (p. 213).

In addition to these experiences described above, Blanton identifies three particular skills which come about from quietening the mind through the addition of time for silence and contemplation:

1 Defusion (as opposed to cognitive fusion): recognizing that an event and our thoughts and perceptions of that event are two different things
2 Acceptance: looking at something without judgment or evaluation, which is similar to a Buddhist notion of detachment/non-attachment, or 'cool' attachment
3 Contact: similar to acceptance, allowing oneself to just experience whatever is happening in the present moment

I have described these skills and attitudes in chapter two as I discussed mindfulness, contemplation, and critical reflection, yet it is interesting to see Blanton also drawing upon similar descriptions as he argues for the benefits of integrating them into narrative practices. He says, the ability to "experience the present moment just as it is [through contemplation…] allows one to 'let go of the past and future and wakeup to what we are now, in this moment'" (Blanton, 2007, p. 215).

Specifically related to the benefits of adding contemplation to narrative practices, Blanton suggests the following:

1 Stories are "just stories. Stories create people, but people also create stories. It is liberating to discover that stories, since they are social constructions, can be discarded for new stories, if the person so desires" (Blanton, 2007, p. 216)
2 "Space develops between the story and the person. In contemplation, people learn to step back from thoughts and see that they are not their thoughts" (Blanton, 2007, p. 216), and so people can step back from their story also
3 People can experience the present moment. "Narrative therapy points us towards the importance of experience, and narrative therapy reminds us that many of our experiences are unnoticed and discarded [...] Contemplation helps people wake up to the experience of the present moment [...] which can become the raw material [or the unique outcomes] for creating new stories" (Blanton, 2007, p. 216)

Indeed, Blanton highlights that integrating contemplation into narrative therapy allows for an experience with the transcendent dimension "that goes beyond one's limited understanding of who one is" (p. 217), and he suggests this draws upon "the language of the soul" (p. 218). He goes on to present a model of psychotherapy that he suggests would be a contemplative-based approach to narrative therapy. For him, this involves interactions "with the soul or divine" (p. 218) in the therapy session. This means discussing the sacred and the holy alongside discussions regarding, family, friends, colleagues, and neighbors, for example. He then suggests this will result in more robust and complex stories for a person since the stories would incorporate experiences that occur within contemplation. I agree with Blanton that all of this is possible with narrative practices, but I do not see the need to develop a new model of psychotherapy. I do not want to argue for a new approach or model of psychotherapy but do see the benefit of incorporating the language of the soul into narrative practices, which will then also open space and time for contemplation, and a respect for the various layers (tentatively understood) and experiences of a person.

Several times as I have been engaged in writing this book, the final prayer after communion in the Anglican Book of Alternative Services has come to mind: "Glory to God, whose power, working in us, can do infinitely more than we can ask or imagine. Glory to God from generation to generation, in the Church and in Christ Jesus, for ever and ever. Amen" (https://www.anglican.ca/wp-content/uploads/BAS.pdf, p. 214). That we can do more than we can possibly ask or imagine was a phrase that particularly resonated for me on my first silent retreat with the Sisters of St. John the Divine, whom I mentioned in the Introduction. As explained, I was staying in the Sisters' guest wing for a silent weekend retreat so that I could work on my PhD dissertation, which felt overwhelming at that point. I suppose I needed to hear reassurance at that time that I could accomplish more than I could imagine, and so the phrase jumped out at me. However, regardless of whether someone has a religious faith, something about this prayer seems to stick in my mind and has me considering everyone I meet as being far more complex, and possible of accomplishing far more, than either I or they can imagine.

Even though language and stories are crucial aspects of narrative practice, I have begun to think about the ways of knowing, and types of wisdom within silence that are difficult to express in words in the therapeutic setting – they are difficult to ask about or imagine. In addition to this, and despite the importance of stories from the past on the development of stories in the future, I wonder how to best explore whether there are possibilities within each present moment which too easily might go unnoticed. Much of therapy will focus on the storied identity of the person consulting us, but sometimes people will want to talk about more than that: Those layer(s) of themselves that are harder to put into words. Therefore, I have begun to more regularly ask people near the end of a counseling session, if there has been something missing from the session, or something that they have not said because it is hard to explain in words. Have I not asked them something they wish I had? I might ask, "If we were to slow down and you were to take a few deep breaths, what story might you tell about this present moment?", or I might say, "You seemed moved by something then, could you describe what was going on?" Unfortunately, this approach continues to rely on language for the response but is one way of acknowledging there is more going on than is always put into words. In fact, I recently suggested to Vicky that not being able to answer a question easily is often a good sign that it was maybe a useful question that is touching upon an area that she has not thought about and processed into language yet. A willingness to sit in silence and acknowledge that something is being experienced anew or for the first time, might certainly aid in movement toward the 'possible to know' and toward 'preferred storylines', to use the language of narrative therapy.

Conclusion

In the introduction to this chapter, I suggested that integrating the language of the soul into narrative practices might aid in supporting 'human flourishing'. Gaye (2010), arguing that Aristotle "explained that the purpose of life is earthly flourishing" (p. 1), suggests "human flourishing can encompass a wide variety of moral and ethical pursuits" (p. 1), not limited to individual well-being but also involving community engagement. He states this type of flourishing is only possible when people access all their potentialities to pursue their freely chosen values. I believe being open to the possibility of those aspects of human life which are perhaps only hinted at in the surfaces of life will provide wider options for human flourishing. For narrative practitioners to be truly open to all these possibilities will involve them being willing to consider the language of the soul as including both the transcendent and the immanent.

In this book, I have explored the theoretical foundations of narrative therapy, which historically have not included a description of either spirituality or the soul. I have argued that this 'gap' may be filled by considering what Teresa of Avila and Edith Stein offer regarding their understanding of the soul. Their descriptions of the soul are complex, suggesting the soul is embodied and yet also offering the possibility of a relationship with the transcendent. Drawing upon Merleau-Ponty and Bakhtin's work further stresses the complexity of the body-soul-world relationship. I believe that many of the conceptions I have presented can easily enrich the theory and practice of narrative therapy, although other aspects of their descriptions may not fit as comfortably with non-spiritual/ secular narrative practitioners. In this chapter I have argued for the need to engage with these ideas I have presented in a dialogic manner, so, in order to 'practice what I preach', the next, concluding, chapter offers a dialogue between myself and David Crawley about which ideas in this book have resonated the most for us, how we have learned from working together on this project, and where we might imagine our thinking will take us next.

Notes

1 http://www.public-domain-poetry.com/william-butler-yeats/aedh-wishes-for-the-cloths-of-heaven-99
2 Interestingly, I recently have had the opportunity to assist in the creation of a creative writing group for people with a cancer diagnosis. This group was developed in collaboration with medical students with training in narrative medicine, a social work student with training in narrative therapy, a local agency which provides supports to people with cancer and myself, as a consultant. The group was offered over six weeks, for two hours each week. Each week's session offered writing prompts informed by narrative therapy's curiosity in preferred or alternative storylines, using a combination of questions, reflections, and visual images, and provided 20 minutes each week for group members to creatively write. This was then followed by time to share or discuss their writing. Although spirituality was not a focus of any of the prompts, several group participants did raise how important their spirituality was to them through their cancer journey.
3 All names and identifying details of clients and case examples have been changed throughout this book.

References

Béres, L. (Ed.) (2017). *Practicing spirituality: Reflecting on meaning-making in personal and professional contexts.* Palgrave MacMillan.

Blanton, P. G. (2007). Adding silence to stories: Narrative therapy and contemplation. *Contemporary Family Therapy, 29*, 211–221. DOI: 10.1007/s1059-007-9047-x

Burack-Weiss, A. (2017). Introduction: Many ways of knowing. In Burack-Weiss,

A., Lawrence, L. S., & Bamat Mijangos, L. (Eds). *Narrative in social work practice: The power and possibility of story* (pp. 1–11). Columbia University Press.

Burack-Weiss, A., Lawrence, L. S., & Bamat Mijangos, L. (Eds). (2017). *Narrative in social work practice: The power and possibility of story*. Columbia University Press.

Charon, R. (2006). *Narrative medicine: Honoring the stories of illness*. Oxford University Press.

Charon, R. (2017). Foreword. In Burack-Weiss, A., Lawrence, L. S., & Bamat Mijangos, L. (Eds). *Narrative in social work practice: The power and possibility of story* (pp. IX–XII). Columbia University Press.

Crawley, D. (2016). Authority in spiritual direction conversations: Dialogic perspectives, *Journal for the Study of Spirituality*, *6*(1), 6–19.

Daly, L., Fahey-McCarthy, E., & Timmins, F. (2019). The experience of spirituality from the perspective of people living with dementia: A systematic review and meta-synthesis. *Dementia*, *18*(2), 448–470. DOI: 10.1177/1471301216680425.

Finlay, L. (2009) Debating phenomenological research methods. *Phenomenology and Practice*, *3*(1), 6–25.

Freeman, J., Epston, D., & Lobovits, D. (1997). *Playful approaches to serious problems: Narrative therapy with children and their families*. W. W. Norton.

Gaye, T. (2010). Editorial: In what ways can reflective practice enhance human flourishing?. *Reflective Practice: International and Multidisciplinary Perspectives*, *11*(1), 1–7.

Guilfoyle, M. (2014). *The person in narrative therapy: A post-structuralist, Foucauldian account*. Palgrave Macmillan.

Hall, J., Mitchell, G., Webber, C., & Johnson, K. (2018). Effects of horticultural therapy on wellbeing among dementia day care programme participants: A mixed-methods study (Innovative practice). *Dementia*, *17*(5), 611–620. DOI: 10.1177/1471301216643847.

Kearney, R. (2016). God after God: An anatheist attempt to reimagine God. In R. Kearney & J. Zimmerman (Eds). *Reimaging the sacred: Richard Kearney debates God* (pp. 6–18). Columbia University Press.

Kearney, R., & Zimmerman, J. (Eds). (2016). *Reimaging the sacred: Richard Kearney debates God*. Columbia University Press.

Sawicki, M. (2000). Editor's Introduction. In M. Sawicki (Ed.) (M. C. Baseheart and M. Sawicki, Trans.). *Philosophy of psychology and the humanities* (pp. XI–XXIII). ICS Publications.

Smith-Carrier, T., Béres, L., Johnson, K., Blake, C., & Howard, J. (2019). Digging into the experiences of therapeutic gardening for people with dementia: An interpretative phenomenological analysis, *Dementia*, *0*(0), 1–18. DOI: 10.1177/1471301219869121

Stein. E. (2000). *Philosophy of psychology and the humanities*. M. Sawicki (Ed.). (M. C. Baseheart and M. Sawicki, Trans.). ICS Publications. (Original work published in 1922.)

Stein, E. (2002). *Finite and eternal being: An attempt at an ascent to the meaning of being*. (K. F. Reinhardt, Trans.). ICS Publications. (Original work published in 1949.)

Stein, E. (2018). *The Science of the Cross*. (J. Koeppel, O.C.D., Trans.). ICS Publications. (Original work published in 1983.)

Teresa of Avila (2013). *Interior Castle* (E. Allison Peers, Trans. & Ed.). Random House. (Original work published in 1577.)

Tyler, P. (2013). *Teresa of Avila: Doctor of the soul*. Bloomsbury.

Tyler, P. (2016). *The pursuit of the soul: Psychoanalysis, soul-making and the Christian tradition*. Bloomsbury T & T Clark.

White, M. (1995). *Re-authoring lives: Interviews and essays*. Dulwich Centre Publications.

White, M. (1997). *Narratives of therapists' lives*. Dulwich Centre Publications.

White, M. (2000). *Reflections on narrative practices: Essays and interviews*. Dulwich Centre Publications.

White, M., & Epston, D. (1990). *Narrative means to therapeutic ends*. W.W. Norton.

Williams, R. (1991). *Teresa of Avila*. Morehouse.

9 Concluding Reflections: A Dialogue on the Language of the Soul for Narrative Practices

Laura Béres and David Crawley

Laura: In chapter three, I commented that Plato wrote about what he learned from, and with, Socrates in the form of *dialogues*. In chapter seven, David drew upon Bakhtin's work and the importance of *dialogic* engagement. In the last chapter I relied upon the idea of *dialogue* between narrative medicine and narrative therapy, and between theists and atheists when 'reimaging the sacred' and considering God after the death of God in secular contexts. It, therefore, seems appropriate to finish this book and the exploration of the language of the soul in dialogue. It would be incongruent *not* to engage in dialogue since David has been willing to contribute to this book and we now have the opportunity to chat about the process of working together and immersing ourselves in the ideas we have presented.

As was described in the Introduction, David and I have each come to this project from slightly different past experiences. I was first a narrative therapist and then became interested in spirituality, the language of the soul, and in potentially moving into providing spiritual direction in the future, whereas David was first a spiritual director and then later took training in narrative therapy. In 2018, David and I had the good fortune of being able to attend the joint 6th European Conference on Religion, Spirituality and Health, and the 5th International Conference of the (then) British Association for the Study of Spirituality, in Coventry, England. We were able to find the time to talk about the possibility of this book, and although we were both excited about the ideas we would present, we were both also cautious, realizing that for many practitioners already committed to narrative practices there could very well be a hesitancy about considering the language of the soul. I am hopeful that we have presented our ideas in an invitational rather than impositional manner. However, before we reflect on the ideas which have resonated most for us, I am curious about what it has been like for you, David, to be involved in this project.

DOI: 10.4324/9781003137450-13

David: The short answer is, I have loved it! Thank you again for the opportunity to offer my thoughts on Bakhtin as a way forward in my quest to find ways of thinking and speaking about the soul, without losing the creativity and fluidity of the social constructionist perspectives on identity that inform narrative practice. As I read what you have written, it strikes me that the work of this book – developing a language of the soul for narrative therapy – is a 'taken-for-granted' in my spiritual direction community. If part of your challenge is the hesitancy which some narrative practitioners may experience around soul language, my challenge is the reverse: helping spiritual directors see that a narrative approach, including its use of postmodern perspectives on personhood, is compatible with the work of being a 'soul friend'. Part of our narrative training is being willing to re-examine what is taken for granted, and one of the gifts of engaging with your work here has been the opportunity to revisit my language and assumptions around the soul, and spirituality more generally. I have encountered old friends, including the desert fathers and mothers, Benedict of Nursia, Teresa of Avila, and John of the Cross, and practices close to the heart of spiritual directors, such as silence and Christian contemplation. Meeting these familiar traditions in a new context and reflecting on the connections you have offered with broader understandings of spirituality and the work of Stein, Merleau-Ponty, and Kearney, as well as with narrative practice, has been hugely stimulating and enriching. All kinds of intertextualities are fizzing in my brain!

One of the new thoughts that I have earmarked for further reflection is Kearney's notion of anatheism. Reading what you had to say about this in chapter eight took me to a Māori whakatauki (proverb) which I read recently. It reflects the importance of voyaging and migration in Māori history. The translation is, "Seek to bring distant horizons closer; sustain and cherish those that have been attained" (Te Pae Tawhiti, 2016). That offers a good description of what is happening for me as I engage with your work. Creating space for language(s) of the soul enables me, as a spiritual director, to cherish familiar shores; at the same time, I experience a call to explore more distant horizons, in terms of conceptualization and practice.

Laura: I very much appreciate this Māori whakatauki you have shared. I like this idea of continuing to cherish what is dear – what I have experienced as ethical and helpful ways of engaging with narrative practices – while I also look for ways of bringing other ideas closer through exploration and dialogue. Sometimes when I present in classroom contexts and conferences on the concept of migration of identity and the notion of liminality, I use a photo of a canoe setting forth across a wide body of water as an image for the feeling of setting sail into the unknown. The metaphor of journey and fluidity are called upon with this image and aligns with the Māori whakatauki. My hope is that all the ideas we have explored in this book should be considered as more fluid and dialogic, rather than considered static or dogmatic. As discussed in relation to anatheism, rigid concepts of God, the Divine, and the soul, can be problematic, and can result in judgement and monologic, instead of dialogic, encounters.

As I look back to the start of my interest in the language of the soul, I realize that at that point in my journey I had a vague but unexamined notion of the soul as probably being different from the body, or perhaps something like the center of myself. I needed to bracket those ideas, and hold onto them lightly, in order to be open to new ways of thinking about the soul as I immersed myself in the literature and attempted to further develop my own contemplative practices. My ideas about the soul and my narrative practices have evolved, through incorporating the contributions of Teresa of Avila and Edith Stein. I began to think of the soul and body as interwoven and layered, with a complex type of center, more like a gateway opening up to something beyond any concept of an individualized self. Actively listening to my former student, Natashia (chapter six), I was reminded of Maurice Merleau-Ponty, whose work has further expanded my ideas, and provided language in relation to 'flesh' and 'chiasma'. I have found it fascinating to see some of the ancient Greek ideas, like 'World soul' (*nous*), resonate with ideas I have cherished, like those from Celtic spirituality about the spark of the Divine in all things and the interweaving of the spiritual and the sacred, which I then also experience as congruent with Merleau-Ponty's work. This certainly adds a further layer of richness to the traditional social work notion of 'person-in-environment'.

Your contributions regarding Bakhtin's work on dialogue and unfinalizability have added further insights, as has the wisdom of the many people with whom I have spoken in counseling contexts. Perhaps we could talk a little about how we see these ideas impacting our practice in narrative therapy and in spiritual direction. What might we have missed if we had not been considering the language of the soul? Why don't you begin, David?

David: I resonate with your descriptions of soul and body as interwoven, rather than separate, and with the wider picture of a world permeated by the sacred. One of my ways of thinking about spirituality is captured in the title of Norman Maclean's novel, *A River Runs Through It*, which begins, "In our family, there was no clear line between religion and fly fishing" (1989, p. 1). So, my equivalent to what you have referred to as the "spark of the Divine in all things," in Celtic spirituality, is the idea of a river of life running through it all. Sometimes we catch a glimpse of it, or experience it, while in spiritually dry times it seems to have gone deep underground. I also like your idea of the soul as being a gateway to something beyond the individualized self – an aspect of human awareness perhaps, through which we find ourselves connected to that mysterious river of life.

That novel may have come to mind because of a recent conversation I had with John,[1] who is passionate about fly fishing. For most of his 80 years, he has not had an active interest in religion or spirituality. Following a recent serious illness, he has become more reflective. Earlier this year, John was fishing in an area of the country that was new to him and found himself overwhelmed by the grandeur and beauty of the landscape. It was, for him, an undeniably spiritual experience, and it sparked a desire to explore what place the divine might have in his remaining years. Talking about such events is not unusual in spiritual direction, but I am aware that people who have experiences like John's are often hesitant to talk about them with others, because they are uncertain of how they will be received (Hawker, 2000).

This is my round about way of responding to your question as to what we might miss if we are not open to, or curious about, the place of the soul in narrative conversations. My feeling is that if we are collaborating with people in listening for hints of hope which have the potential to be sustaining and grow into alternative stories, then an openness to matters of the soul is important. That certainly includes White's 'little sacraments of daily existence', but, in my experience, it can also include making room in a conversation for silence and stillness, within which people can recover forgotten knowledges or memories, or find themselves quietly aware of an unlooked-for source of hope or reassurance – an echo of the river of life. A few days ago, in a spiritual direction session, Peter reflected on his recurring experience of being visited by fears. At his suggestion, we finished the session with five minutes of prayerful silence, during which he sensed a divine voice saying simply, 'Don't be afraid'. Cognitively, Peter was already aware that he had no reason to be fearful. In the silence, however, he experienced these words as being addressed not only to his rational mind, but to his soul. I wonder, Laura, might we extend Michael White's idea of 'double listening' to include a contemplative quality of listening, on the part of the practitioner and/or the client, as part of our practice? How do we tune our ears to soul language?

Laura: What a great question! I think my initial reaction is that we at least should not ignore people's use of the word 'soul'. Being curious about what a person means by this and what is implied by it can open up a range of conversations that might otherwise be missed. As Holloway (2007) has suggested, "patients [feel] inhibited in expressing spiritual and existential concerns with non-religious professionals" (p. 273), pointing out that this can seriously impede practitioners in engaging in conversations regarding spirituality or the 'soul' – even missing when referrals to spiritual or religious professionals might be appreciated. Finding ways to be comfortable and competent with spirituality and the language of the soul is the first step and does not even need the skill of double listening at this point. Some people will raise 'soul' directly, as Lydia did when she said she needed to 'feed her soul somehow – and that walking in nature often helped' (chapter one), and yet others may raise this sort of hunger in an 'absent but implicit' manner. On the one hand, Lydia spoke clearly about her soul and spirituality while Jane (also in chapter one) spoke clearly and directly about her fundamentalist religious faith. On the other hand, Eve (chapter six) indicated having a 'highly personalized and individualized' form of spirituality and a preference for speaking about 'true Self' rather than her soul and Vicky (chapter eight) said that although she had been taken to church as a child, she had now lost all hope and believed she had only been born to suffer and then die. With Lydia, Jane, Eve, and Vicky, I found it most useful to trust the frameworks of narrative conversations as well as concepts related to the language of the soul. Just recently, Vicky was telling me about a couple of events that had happened during the two weeks since we had last spoken (events in the recent history in the landscape of action in a reauthoring conversation). It seemed as though these events and her reactions to them were part of the problem storyline and reminded her of experiences of abuse from her ex-husband. I took the chance that asking questions that placed them within that storyline might decrease their impact when she could see them as part of that storyline and separate from what she had previously indicated was her preferred storyline: one of hope that might have links to events in her more distant personal history with her mother. Double listening means listening to the problem storyline at the same time as I am listening for opportunities to move into the preferred storyline, as well as listening for what is implied in her statements of hopelessness – that she has had experiences of hope against which she may be comparing her current feelings. In adding the language of the soul to my engagement with people, including Vicky, I sense I am seeing even more layers to people and their experiences. I am interested in engaging with people regarding their thoughts, feelings, and behaviors, as I make use of the narrative maps (White, 2007), but now there is also more room for being curious about what occurs in silence, wondering about people's intuition, and all the various 'layers' of their embodied soul. As discussed in relation to anatheism, I think this makes room for bringing the secular into the sacred and the sacred into the secular. For those who are more spiritual and religious, and here I am particularly thinking of Jane, mentioned above and in chapter one, there is also room for the transcendent. Jane, for instance, talked about her image of God as being rather authoritarian and judgmental. In deconstructing her ideas of God, she began to think that she had imposed her experiences of authoritarian parents onto her image of a father-God-figure. In considering other images of parents and other images of God, she moved into a position of considering her God as more like a loving and supportive parent or friend. This had a corresponding effect on her sense of herself as a parent. She had told me that her sense of identity was very much tied to her image of herself as a good parent, and yet, over the course of our counseling appointments, she also reported becoming less controlling in her parenting.

I've now touched on a couple of ideas that I think are of interest to you: ways of knowing and the transcendent. Perhaps you could let me know if I have gone too far off track from your question, if anything resonated, or where this has now taken your thinking.

David: There is much that resonates here! Your quote from Holloway, concerning the inhibition people can feel in talking about "spiritual and existential concerns" with non-religious professionals reminds me of some work I did around experiences of the "continued presence" of lost loved ones (Crawley, 2019). I found researchers in this field suggesting that while such experiences are not uncommon, people in western contexts often find it difficult to talk about them in therapeutic conversations. I can appreciate that on the part of practitioners, too, there may be discomfort when it comes to talking about spiritual issues. That might be due to unfamiliarity with the area, or to cultural and psychological discourses which invite skeptical or pathologizing responses to stories such as the continued presence of a lost loved one, hearing God's voice, or a sense of oneness with the Divine/the universe. I therefore resonate with what you say about finding ways to be 'comfortable and competent with spirituality and the language of the soul', and making room in our interactions with people for all that has significance for them, including all the 'layers' of their embodied souls.

During my narrative therapy training, I found James and Melissa Griffith's (2003) book *Encountering the Sacred in Psychotherapy: How to Talk to People about Their Spiritual Lives* a helpful resource. In their own practice, they prefer not to raise direct questions about spirituality, "unless we have a sense that these questions make sense within the language and culture of the person" (p. 46). Instead, they adopt a stance of curiosity which includes asking existential questions which have the potential to open a hospitable space for talk of spirituality or the soul, should that be helpful. Examples of these questions (p. 46) are What has sustained you?; From what sources do you draw strength in order to cope?; Where do you find peace?; What is your clearest sense of the meaning of your life at this time?

As someone who may be *too* ready to bring the scared into the secular, I find this broader approach a respectful and helpful way forward. In spiritual direction, I sometimes find myself moving in the reverse direction, that is, inviting people to bring more of the secular into the sacred. Religious discourses can find expression in rather generalized resolutions to have more faith, hope, or love. In those instances, I might ask curious questions about the *embodied* aspects of such an intention, bearing in mind the soul-body-world connections discussed in this book. I might ask where in the person's life the spiritual quality of love, say, has turned up in their past actions, as well as how, in practical terms, they imagine it might become a greater part of their life and relationships in the future (landscape of action).

When it comes to ways of knowing, I am aware that narrative therapy is sometimes criticized for being too intellectual. In chapter eight, you reflected on a time when you may have 'overly privileged cognitive elements' within your practice, including definitions of spirituality which focused mainly on meaning and purpose. It was interesting to read about the research you and others did into what attracted people with dementia to a therapeutic gardening program, and how this deepened your appreciation of the need for 'more than just rational exploration'. You then described the value of incorporating connection to nature, contemplation, and silence into narrative practices. I would add to these being open to what might be gained by paying attention to the body, intuitive 'hunches', dreams, or the imagination, or by engagement in creative activities. During my PhD research, I found that embodied, intuitive, and spiritual forms of knowledge played an important role in participants' acts of resistance to unhelpful practices of religious authority. I also noticed that most of the women I interviewed reported that their embodied and intuitive ways of knowing were at best discounted, and at worst labeled as dangerous, by their religious leaders (Crawley, 2014, p. 239). That seems to fit with Davies' (1991) suggestion that assertions of the rational over the irrational, and the conscious over the unconscious, are expressions of humanist and masculinist discourse.

I have said more than enough for now, Laura, but that last point evokes the ethical and political intentions reflected in narrative therapeutic practice. For you, how does that stance connect with the language of the soul?

Laura: I also appreciate the Griffiths' work; your reference to them and the helpful suggestions regarding questions that can be used remind me of Canda and Furman's (1999) work: *Spiritual Diversity in Social Work Practice: The Heart of Helping*. Not only do they discuss spirituality in all its complexity, providing suggestions as to how

> practitioners can prepare themselves for the inclusion of spirituality in their work, decide on the appropriateness of raising spirituality with someone, and then assess for the impacts of spirituality, they also provide an extensive list of examples of spiritually oriented helping activities that can be used in practice with individuals, families, groups, organizations, and communities (pp. 292–293). These activities range from engaging the active imagination, using art and dance, care for the body, guided visualizations, and mindfulness, to participating in nature retreats, and yoga. Merely asking about whether a person is engaged in any of these practices is a simple way of assessing a person's interest in spirituality. I would be comfortable adding some of these activities into my practice in a therapy office, while others might just be offered as ideas someone might want to explore outside of counseling. These activities appear to align with the complexity of the language of the soul – considering the body-soul-world relationship – with activities being offered in all the various elements of the soul. I was thinking about this language of layers, or elements, of the soul as I was walking my dog this morning.

After a few hours at my computer, I was drawn to go for a neighborhood walk with my dog, Biscuit. I have started to trust my intuition more over the years and if part of me thinks it is time to take a walk, I will usually heed this advice. I attempt to walk mindfully, letting my thoughts come and go rather than overly focusing on any particular idea. I had been thinking, before my walk, that I was not completely comfortable with the word 'layers' in relation to the soul, and as I was walking this came back to me simply and passed by in my mind as I realized I would merely point this out when I came back to my computer and this dialogue. I have used this term as Teresa of Avila did in her descriptions of mansions within the interior castle of her soul, and as Stein used it in relation to elements of a human being in her earlier work. The challenge with the word is that it implies a depth of layers – one over the other – which then can conjure up the image of digging for a certain depth of understanding or meaning. When I was a beginning social worker, I remember the image of layers of an onion being used frequently to suggest the need to peel the various layers of the emotional onion away in order to access the innermost emotion, suggesting that *it* was the most important – anger was often described as the outer layer sometimes covering up an emotional hurt, for instance. I wonder whether speaking of elements or aspects of the soul might move us away from a hierarchy, or whether just thinking of a multifaceted soul might be useful. I suppose, alternatively, it might be best to hold on to any of these terms tentatively. As I initially said, any term that becomes inflexible runs the risk of becoming dogmatic and shutting down dialogue.

That was a fairly long description of my concerns about the idea of 'layers' but hopefully, also, an example of a simple way of incorporating a recognition of intuition and a physical activity such as walking with animals, which for many of us involves elements of spirituality and responding to various aspects of the soul. This leads me to your question about ethical and political intentions of narrative therapy. I might speak of these intentions as related to social justice. In social work in North America, social work contains a range of possible practice focusses: individual, couple, family, and group counseling, as well as child welfare work (micro); community engagement, advocacy and practice (mezzo); and policy and government-related work (macro). This fits within the social work commitment to think of the 'person in environment', as I mentioned earlier. (Zapf [2007; 2010] has argued that this needs to be expanded in practice to include the physical environment as well as the social and cultural context, which is consistent with how some of Merleau-Ponty's work has been taken up, as described in chapter six.) And, when I think about the soul, I think about interiority (such as the *via negativa* and apophatic prayer, as discussed in chapter two) balanced with the call to act in socially just manners in the world – thinking again of the image of both Mary and Martha that I mentioned in the last chapter. This might resonate with the idea of some of us being more introverted and some more extroverted, some called to micro social work and others to macro. I think it is all important, and perhaps the mix is just a little different for each of us. By introducing the language of the soul to narrative practices I am not suggesting interiority is now the preferred agenda – I am hoping it adds further richness and complexity alongside the ethical and political commitments.

My comments have become even longer! I wonder what might have interested you in what I've said, and I also think we should perhaps turn our attention to our next steps. You've mentioned earmarking Kearney's work on anatheism for further reflection, but is there anything else that has captured your interest? How do we keep hold of all these ideas lightly and what possibilities might open up by doing so?

David: Your reflections on taking a mindful walk with Biscuit remind me of how important I find it to take long walks whenever I spend time on retreat. Some years ago, after a difficult personal crisis, I went on an eight-day silent retreat at St. Beuno's Ignatian retreat center in North Wales. I began the retreat feeling that my soul was not in great shape, and my instinct was to walk every day in the hills, despite the freezing December weather. The physical effort of walking and feeling the icy wind and rain on my face felt like an important embodied spiritual practice. Paradoxically, those bracing winter walks worked a steady thaw in my soul, and I ended the retreat more at peace with where my life was heading. Picking up on your hesitancy about reifying the language of 'layers', for me

> that retreat was not a time to peel the layers of the emotional onion, to get to the innermost source of my pain, although there have been occasions when that was an important task. It was engaging my body with the landscape and the weather that brought solace and clarity. So, I like your idea of the soul as being multifaceted, a nexus of elements, rather than a hierarchy of layers. It is hard not to think of Teresa of Avila's mansions in hierarchical terms, and to value the innermost chambers, and interior forms of spirituality, above others. As I think about my own home, I do have a favorite space (my outdoor study where I'm sitting now), but I don't count it as more important than the other rooms or expect that I should spend more time here than anywhere else. Each room is important in its own way, and I move between them as need warrants.

As I think about this now, and about holding all language about the multifaceted aspects of the soul lightly, as you have suggested, I experience a tangible sense of freedom and spaciousness. I don't need to choose between being Mary or Martha! Interiority and exteriority need not be in competition. You cited a lovely phrase from Catherine Keller in the previous chapter: "there is a chiasmus between apophatic interiority and kataphatic outreach into action". I see each aspect of that chiasmus enriching the other. I own the fact that I have a quiet and reflective personality which inclines me more toward apophatic interiority – no wonder my study is my favorite room in the house! I am therefore grateful to others whose commitment to kataphatic outreach calls me beyond my comfortable interior space toward engagement in social justice. At the same time, as a spiritual director, I sometimes find myself inviting those whose lives are full of outward action to consider spending some time in rest and reflection; not as an escape from the ethical demands of life in the world, but as a way of resourcing themselves to meet those demands and to discern what is most important.

In terms of next steps for me, alongside the idea of anatheism, this book poses a question which I feel I need to sit with some more: How might the language of soul contribute to an improvement of relationship between human beings and our physical environment? It is a pertinent question, in light of historical dualisms between body/world and soul, which you have noted. Over against those dualisms you have traced a unitive theme. In chapter two, for example, you touched on Plato's idea of a 'World soul' (*nous*) which is reflected in the individual soul's intelligence. You also mentioned in that chapter the ways in which humans and the physical world are interconnected within various Indigenous spiritualities. The collective grief which Māori, the Indigenous people of Aotearoa New Zealand, express in relation to the loss of their lands through colonization testifies to the inseparability for them of land, ancestry, spirituality, and identity. In the conclusion to chapter six, you suggested that Merleau-Ponty's idea of the "shared fabric (or flesh) of this world […] requires, in therapeutic practices, spiritual direction or pastoral counseling, a commitment to remembering the body-mind-world relationship", and you go to on to connect this with the language of soul. I catch glimpses of what this means for me personally and for my spiritual direction practice, but, in terms of the whakatauki cited earlier, it feels like a horizon which is still more distant from my lived experience than I would like. Globally, the climate change crisis and the pandemic which the world is facing make it imperative for me to work at bringing this horizon closer. Where are the next steps for you Laura?

Laura: My next steps are so similar to yours that I feel I could just say, 'ditto' and conclude this dialogic chapter right here! The rapid spread of COVID-19 around the world dramatically highlighted our interconnectedness, as did the World Health Organization's comments that no one is safe from COVID until we are all vaccinated – not just the people in affluent countries!

Here in North America as in New Zealand, Indigenous communities are grieving due to the ongoing effects of colonization. In addition to this in Canada, Indigenous communities are also grieving due to the recent discovery of unmarked graves of hundreds of Indigenous children who were forced into residential schools, the last one of which only finally closed as recently as 1996 (www.thecanadianencyclopedia.ca/en/article/residential-schools). The "Indian Residential School Settlement Agreement", in 2007, established processes for claiming financial compensation for survivors of the schools, and also established The Truth and Reconciliation Commission (TRC) (https://www.rcaanc-cirnac.gc.ca/eng/). The TRC traveled across Canada meeting with over 6,500 witnesses between 2007 and 2015. In the TRC's final meeting in Ottawa in June 2015, 94 calls to action were presented, to continue to facilitate reconciliation. Progress has been very slow in relation to these calls to action, which has been highlighted alongside the recent discovery of the unmarked graves. The Canadian government and the religious organizations that ran the residential schools and everyone else in Canada as witnesses to this system and ongoing effects of the system are called upon to educate themselves about the history of colonization and the residential schools as well as commit to working for reconciliation. This involves external, kataphatic outreach and action, as we have described it above – not just a withdrawal into interiority.

In North America, at the same time as we are called to acknowledge the effects of colonization on Indigenous communities, the Black Lives Matter movement has brought to heightened attention, after the murder of George Floyd in the USA, the need to use critical race theory to examine the manner in which race impacts the lives of all people of color. I have been integrating critical race theory into the critical perspectives lens of critical reflection on practice as I teach this model to social work students, but this is only one small step in a much broader system that requires change. In my immediate community, a Muslim family was murdered by a hit and run driver who indicated he had purposefully targeted them due to their faith. An outpouring of support and allyship was demonstrated by members of interfaith and nonfaith organizations, with thousands of people marching through the city from the site of the crime to the Mosque which the family had attended. Speeches and commitments were made by local and federal politicians and community members to work toward change so this would never happen again. Many front gardens in the city hold signs reading, 'Love over Hate' and 'No matter where you are from, you are welcome', and yet so much more still needs to be done.

As we have been writing this concluding dialogue, the Taliban has taken over Afghanistan and we've seen pictures on news broadcasts of the desperation in the Kabul airport as people attempt to leave the country; there has been an earthquake resulting in devastation, loss of life, and injuries in Haiti; wildfires are out of control in the western provinces of Canada, in Greece and Turkey, as dry weather and extreme heat have resulted in the perfect condition for fires, with many people required to evacuate their home towns, and not always having a home to return to. 'Thoughts and prayers' is a phrase witnesses will often use to let people know they are thinking of them in their times of trouble, but thoughts and prayers are only ever a partial response, and, if meaningful, should result in action and change.

A few years ago, I saw the documentary film, *Anthropocene: The Human Epoch* (https://theanthropocene.org/film), in which humanity's impact on the planet is shown to quite frightening effect. I had already been considering how to engage in greater simplicity, and the film added to my concerns. However, with these thoughts as a backdrop, I recently engaged in the process of critical reflection with a group of colleagues (Béres et al., 2022), in which they assisted me in deconstructing and reconstructing my reactions to an experience that occurred during the first lockdown of the pandemic in Canada. In my written description of my experience, I mention watching the livestream of Andrea Bocelli's "Music for Hope" in April 2020, and being struck at the time by the images from cities around the world of empty streets. At that time, social media was sharing images of clearer skies, with lack of air traffic, and being able to see fish in the canals of Venice, which were also clearer with lack of boating. I hoped that one of the side effects of the pandemic might be that the planet would have a chance for some healing as people maybe embraced a simpler life; of course, it is those of us living in the most affluent countries of the world who need to consider simplifying. Now, 16 months later, people seem much more interested in going back to their old 'normal', despite descriptions of needing to think about a 'new normal'.

Although I can find this all quite disheartening at times, as one small part of my next step, I have ordered a copy of Catherine Keller's *Facing Apocalypse: Climate, Democracy, and Other Last Chances* (2021). I am hoping to learn more about how to respond to these last chances individually and collectively. Part of responding collectively, for me, is raising these issues with students. While most of my work involves teaching counseling and critical reflection on practice approaches, I believe I can only teach these approaches as ethical and socially just activities if these broader social, cultural, and environmental contexts are also taken into account. I also believe the language of the soul can help with this project, if we remember the relationship between body-soul-world and the interweaving of the sacred, secular, and natural environment. However, there is always more to learn, reinforcing the need to hold onto our own ideas gently and engage in truly dialogic encounters, especially with those who are asking us to be witnesses and allies.

David: Our conversation has reached a sobering terminus, and I feel the temptation to withdraw into the relative safety of my interior world! But I am encouraged by the lives of people who have been able to hold together a deep commitment both to the life of the soul and the call to action in the world. I am thinking of people like Dorothy Day, Mahatma Gandhi, Thomas Merton, Mother Teresa, and the Dalai Lama. Of these, the one I know best is Thomas Merton, Trappist monk and writer, whose father was a New Zealander. He is widely known for his writings on contemplative practices, but in the last few years of his life he pursued silence and solitude, interreligious dialogue, and peace activism with equal vigor (Forest, 2008). I am drawn to know more of his story, in the hope, once more, that "it is copying that originates" (Geertz in White & Epston, 1990, p. 13).

Thank you again, Laura, for the opportunity to contribute in a small way to this important project, and for the richness of this conversation.

Laura: My pleasure! I hope we will remain in dialogue and that readers also will feel invited to reach out to us to comment and keep the conversation alive.

Note

1 All names and identifying details of clients and case examples have been changed throughout this book.

References

Béres, L., & Baird, S. with contributions from Bedggood, J., Bodkin, K., Britton-deJeu, H., Cadotte, E., Elsie-McKendrick, A., & Roger, D. (2022). Developing and sustaining critical reflection on social work practice. In Fook, J. (Ed.). *Organizing critical reflection: Experiences from social care.* Routledge.

Canda, E. R., & Furnman, L. D. (1999). *Spiritual diversity in social work practice: The heart of helping*. The Free Press.

Crawley, D. R. (2014). *Stories of resistance to religious authority: A discursive analysis*. [Doctoral thesis, The University of Waikato]. The University of Waikato Research Commons. https://hdl.handle.net/10289/8665

Crawley, D. R. (2019). Spiritual care and stories of continued presence: Taking care not to silence the dead. *Journal for the Study of Spirituality*, *9*(1), 6–19. 10.1080/20440243.2019.1581323

Davies, B. (1991). The concept of agency: A feminist post-structuralist analysis. *Postmodern Critical Theorising*, *30*, 42–53.

Forest, J. (2008). *Living with wisdom: A life of Thomas Merton*. Orbis Books.

Griffith, J. L., & Griffith, M. E. (2003). *Encountering the sacred in psychotherapy: How to talk with people about their spiritual lives*. Guilford Press.

Hawker, P. (2000). *Secret affairs of the soul: Ordinary people's extraordinary experiences of the sacred*. Northstone Publishing.

Holloway, M. (2007). Spiritual need and the core business of social work. *British Journal of Social Work*, *37*(2), 265–280.

Keller, C. (2021). *Facing apocolypse: Climate, democracy, and other last chances*. Orbis Books.

Maclean, N. (1989). *A river runs through it*. Pennyroyal Press.

Te Pae Tawhiti. (2016). Retrieved 26 April 2021 from https://www.horizons.govt.nz/HRC/media/Media/Accelerate%2025/Te-Pae-Tawhiti-A4-Booklet-WEB.pdf?ext=

White, M. (2007). *Maps of narrative practice*. W.W. Norton.

White, M., & Epston, D. (1990). *Narrative means to therapeutic ends*. W.W. Norton.

Zapf, M. K. (2007). Profound connections between person and place: Exploring location, spirituality, and social work. In J. Coates, J. R. Graham, B. Swartzentruber, & B. Ouellette (Eds). *Spirituality and social work: Selected Canadian readings* (pp. 229–242). Canadian Scholars Press.

Zapf, M. K. (2010). Social work and the environment: Understanding people and place, *Critical social work*, *11*(3), 30–46.

Index

For Product Safety Concerns and Information please contact our EU
representative GPSR@taylorandfrancis.com
Taylor & Francis Verlag GmbH, Kaufingerstraße 24, 80331 München, Germany

www.ingramcontent.com/pod-product-compliance
Lightning Source LLC
Chambersburg PA
CBHW070330270326
41926CB00017B/3832

* 9 7 8 0 3 6 7 6 8 4 2 2 8 *